MW00680764

The Diabetic Health Journal written by Lauren Bongiorno
Type 1 Diabetes Edition

Published by Emily Page LLC, http://emilyannepage.com/publishing/
January 1, 2018. Inquiries: info@emilyannepage.com

Cover, illustration, and formatting by Kat Reyes Design
http://katreyesdesign.com

Edited by Emma Plehal

The Diabetic Health Journal (Sage)
**Book ISBN-10:** 1-947684-03-4
**Book ISBN-13:** 978-1-947684-03-4

The Diabetic Health Journal (Blush)
**Book ISBN-10:** 1-947684-04-1
**Book ISBN-13:** 978-1-947684-04-1

MSRP: $34.99

# THE DIABETIC HEALTH JOURNAL

## A 3-MONTH GUIDE TO ACHIEVING YOUR BEST A1C

## TYPE 1 DIABETES EDITION
BY LAUREN BONGIORNO, HC

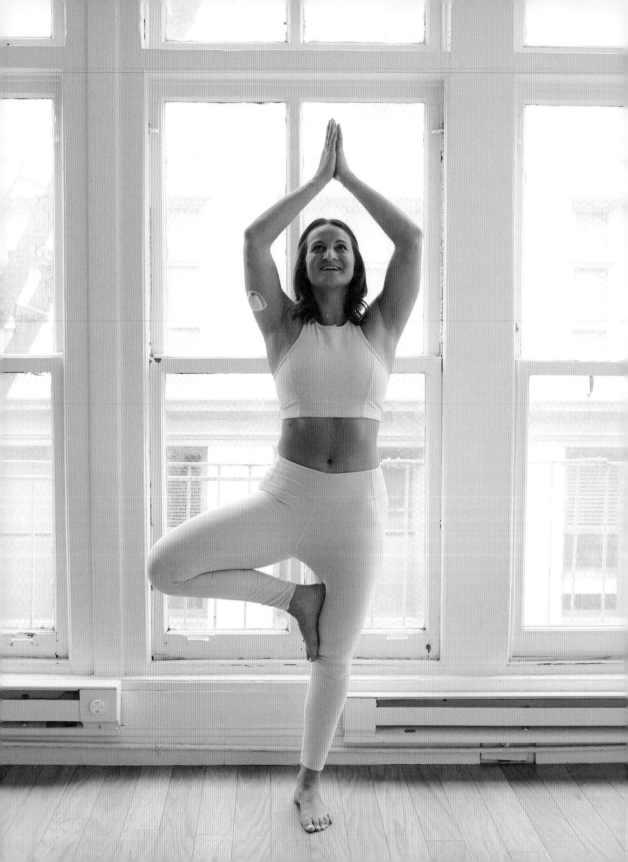

DEAR FRIEND,

Before you dive into this journal, take a deep breath in through your nose and sigh it out through your mouth. Let it all go: Everything you've done or haven't done. Everything you think you should be. Everything you think you should have accomplished by now.

Put all disempowering thoughts in the past so you can clear up space for only what serves you. Then, and only then, will you be able to cultivate positive changes in your mind, body, and soul over these next three months.

This journal is your support and guidance in bridging the gap between where you are and where you want to be. You are worthy, deserving, and capable of achieving it all — we all are.

In the next few pages you'll find an introduction and education section, an outline of how to use the journal, plus self-assessment and goal setting exercises. These exercises are the core of this journal and part of your tools for success. Skipping them is like giving yourself insulin at a meal without knowing your blood sugar first. You'll get the most out of this journal if you start with a solid base without rushing to get to the final destination. Enjoy the journey.

I hope that the tools in this journal will make as much of an impact on your life as they have on mine. I'm looking forward to hearing about all of your progress, so send me an e-mail at info@laurenbongiorno.com. Also, you can connect with me and the journal community through the social channels below.

Always remember, you can be a work in progress and love yourself where you are at the same time.

I BELIEVE IN YOU. WE'RE ALL IN THIS TOGETHER.

*Lauren Bongiorno*

CONNECT WITH ME
INSTAGRAM • @lauren_bongiorno
WEBSITE • www.laurenbongiorno.com

CONNECT WITH #myDHJ TRIBE

INSTAGRAM • @diabetichealthjournal
DECIDE & CONQUER FACEBOOK GROUP • https://www.facebook.com/groups/decideandconquerdiabetes/
WEBSITE • www.diabetichealthjournal.com

# A 360° APPROACH

**THERE IS A GAPING HOLE IN THE WAY WE ARE TAUGHT TO MANAGE OUR DIABETES.** The way the system is set up, we go to the doctor every 3 months, check our A1C, maybe tweak some basal rates, refill our prescriptions and leave with the goal of gaining more control of our blood sugars for next time. Physicians and their team, regardless of how knowledgeable and well intentioned they are, rarely have the time or resources to give every single one of us the individual attention we need not only physically, but mentally and emotionally as well. As a result, many of us struggle in between appointments with a lack of motivation, self-discipline, understanding, routine, or consistency needed to reach our goals. Or maybe you have those under control, but struggle with lack of support, acceptance, balance, or self-love.

One of my favorite thought leaders, Tony Robbins, says to identify your problems, but give power and energy to the solutions. If the problem is that we expect someone else to be responsible for guiding us in all aspects of our lives with diabetes, then I propose a solution in which we take on that responsibility ourselves, listening to our bodies and reflecting on what is working and what needs to change. Besides, at the end of the day, you and I have the potential to know our bodies better than anyone else ever will.

A theme I live my life by is: "Insanity is doing the same thing over and over again and expecting different results." If you aren't achieving the happiness and health you want, you don't have to change your goals, you just have to change your method.

**FOR YEARS AFTER I WAS DIAGNOSED WITH TYPE 1 DIABETES**, I struggled to find the "right" answer to gaining peak control of my blood sugar numbers, my health, and my happiness. I spent years over-exercising, eating low-carb/ high fat, eating high- carb/ low-fat, being anxious around food, going up and down in weight, you name it, i've been there, I get it. I was constantly looking to the outside for answers, yet was consistently feeling overwhelmed, confused, and still, unhappy. When I started practicing yoga, I was introduced to the concept of mindfulness and self-study, which encourages you to examine your behaviors, habits, and patterns. I started to implement this self awareness in all areas of my life and was able to see clearly on my own the changes that needed to be made. It wasn't until I started to incorporate more of a holistic, 360 degree approach that emphasized wellness

> I WAS CONSTANTLY LOOKING TO THE OUTSIDE FOR ANSWERS, YET WAS CONSISTENTLY FEELING OVERWHELMED, CONFUSED, AND STILL, UNHAPPY.
>
> — LNB

> **THE ANSWERS ARE IN SLOWING DOWN, REFLECTING, AND PRIORITIZING OURSELVES ON A HOLISTIC LEVEL.**

throughout the mind, body, and soul, that I found peace and empowerment I had never felt before. I was in control for the first time in my life. Most people look at control as the ability to influence all outcomes, and therefore think that it's impossible to achieve; but in my perspective, I believe control is the ability to influence the outcomes you can, and let go and move on from the ones you cannot. THAT is the type of control I am proposing is possible for all of us.

**AS A DIABETIC HEALTH COACH**, I have worked with hundreds of people with diabetes using this concept. I have been privileged to help clients from all over the world who range in age, occupation, race, and time living with diabetes, yet all of them share similar thoughts when they first reach out to me. They are frustrated, tired, fed up, and anxious for change. They feel like diabetes has completely consumed them, and it is my joy to help them find control and greater happiness in their own life. In almost every instance, my clients' goals are to lower their A1C, achieve more stable and predictable blood sugar numbers, increase insulin sensitivity, increase energy, and have a more positive and balanced mindset around their diabetes. Through working with them and watching them achieve their goals, and in many cases surpass them, I've come to a realization: The answers are in slowing down, reflecting, and prioritizing ourselves on a holistic level. It's about learning to become more proactive than reactive.

I've helped people drop their A1C as drastically as a 12 to a 6.5 over a 6-month period. I've taken people who were scared of carbs and struggling with diabulimia to a place of balance and control that comes from an empowered mindset, rather than a restrictive and fearful one. This is in part due to the various coaching techniques I use and the passion I have for what I do, but even more so from my clients' commitment to putting in the work daily.

**OVER THE NEXT 3 MONTHS, YOU ARE GOING TO TAKE CHARGE OF YOUR LIFE.** You will develop a routine devoted to creating positive habits that will in turn positively affect your blood sugar numbers. When you elevate one area of your life, it helps to raise all the others. Trust me, all it takes is a few extra moments throughout your day to write, reflect, and make little improvements along the way. These little improvements will add up to big change. It might seem tedious to write everything down, especially the blood sugar/food logging, but I promise you life is harder when you don't take the steps to do it. Being "too busy" is a decision. Don't wait for it to be the right time. Create it. Start today knowing that you cannot become your best self or attract into your life all you want unless you are your healthiest self.

**THERE ARE NO COINCIDENCES IN LIFE.** This journal was brought to you to for a reason. By picking it up, you've already conquered the hardest part: initiating change. Now let's flip the page and let's flip the switch.

# EDUCATION

## #1. THE BREAKDOWN

Your A1C is reflective of your average blood sugar over the 3 months prior to blood work. The chart on the following page helps to translate the estimated average glucose your A1C reflects.

## #2. IT'S MORE THAN THE NUMBER

While studies have shown that an A1C below 7.0 significantly lowers your risk for complications, it's important to not get too attached to the number. Keep your A1C goal in the back of your mind and focus your attention on what you will gain along the way as you reach it.

## #3. RAISE THE BAR (OR DROP IT!)

Over time, it's easy to get desensitized to those high, but not "so high" numbers. If you're comfortable sitting around 180 mg/dL (10.1 mmol), remember that a body without diabetes should be between 70 and 120 mg/dL (3.8 and 6.7 mmol). Instead of becoming complacent and accepting of numbers that are "good for a person with diabetes," set the bar high and strive for that tighter range.

## #4. REWARDS TODAY

Whenever someone has said to me, "You want to take care of yourself now so you don't have complications later on in life," I don't find it to be the number one motivator. Most days, I don't see a high blood sugar and think about how that specific number is going to directly affect me 20 years from now. I'm thinking about how crappy I feel and how I don't want to get out of bed. Please don't get me wrong: I'm a total supporter of having my toes and eyesight when I'm 80. Yet, I think it can be motivating for most people to think of the instant gratification we'll receive day to day when we take care of our blood sugars. Such as:

- ✔ Increased mood
- ✔ Increased energy
- ✔ Increased happiness
- ✔ Increased productivity
- ✔ Increased concentration
- ✔ Increased quality of workouts
- ✔ Decreased irritability with children, parents, partner, and friends
- ✔ Increased ability to be more present
- ✔ Boosted libido
- ✔ Decreased anxiety/depression

## #5. WRITING VS. TYPING

Maybe you want to know the science behind journaling and whether it's actually worth putting pen to paper in such a technologically driven society. Studies show that writing stimulates and engages your brain more effectively than typing. Journaling helps you to slow down and practice mindfulness that will translate to your everyday life. In fact, writing by hand requires more subtle and complicated motion from your fingers than typing, so it increases activity in the brain's motor cortex, which is an effect that is actually similar to meditation.

# ESTIMATED AVERAGE GLUCOSE

| A1C | ESTIMATED AVERAGE GLUCOSE (mg/dL) | ESTIMATED AVERAGE GLUCOSE (mmol/L) |
|---|---|---|
| 5% | 97 | 5.4 |
| 5.5% | 111 | 6.2 |
| 6% | 126 | 7.0 |
| 6.5% | 140 | 7.8 |
| 7% | 154 | 8.6 |
| 7.5% | 169 | 9.4 |
| 8% | 183 | 10.1 |
| 8.5% | 197 | 10.9 |
| 9% | 212 | 11.8 |
| 9.5% | 226 | 12.6 |
| 10% | 240 | 13.4 |
| 10.5% | 255 | 14.1 |
| 11% | 269 | 14.9 |
| 11.5% | 283 | 15.7 |
| 12% | 298 | 16.5 |

# JOURNEY INWARD

## SELF ASSESSMENT

*We cannot improve until we know where to improve.*

1. What was your last A1C? _____

2. What is your average fasting blood sugar (waking up)? _____

3. My current basal insulin:

| TIME OF DAY | MY BASAL |
|---|---|
| EXAMPLE: *12:00am* | *.65* |
| | |
| | |
| | |
| | |
| | |
| | |

4. My current Insulin: Carb Ratio/s:

| TIME OF DAY | MY ICR |
|---|---|
| EXAMPLE: *12:00am* | *1:10* |
| | |
| | |
| | |
| | |
| | |
| | |

5. My current Insulin Sensitivity Factor/s:

| TIME OF DAY | MY ISF |
|---|---|
| EXAMPLE: *12:00am* | *1:50* |
| | |
| | |
| | |
| | |
| | |
| | |

6. On a scale from 0-10, rate your happiness in each of the following areas:

_____ a.) Diabetes Management

_____ b.) Exercise

_____ c.) Sleep

_____ d.) Energy

_____ e.) Peace of Mind/Stress and Anxiety Management

_____ f.) Nutrition/Relationship with Food

_____ g.) Relationships with Family, Friends, and Co-Workers

_____ h.) Self Love/Acceptance

7. My target Blood Glucose:

_____

# GOAL SETTING

The DHJ approach to goal-setting is rooted in identifying the small, powerful, incremental improvements each day that will lead to massive change over time. Below you will list three overarching goals you wish to accomplish over the next three months followed by one action step for each.

**Your overarching goals** will be big-picture items you want to accomplish. Examples include lowering your A1C, eating healthier, discovering blood sugar patterns, increasing energy, having fewer out of range blood glucose numbers, or reducing anxiety. **Your action steps** will be the specific tasks or actions you feel you need to implement at this time in order to reach the overarching goal. Making your action steps S.M.A.R.T – Specific, Measurable, Achievable, Realistic, and Time framed will provide you with the most clarity to track and measure your progress. For instance, rather than making your action step "I want to exercise more," you would say, "I will exercise 4x per week for 45 minutes each session." The more clear and explicit you are, the more likely you'll be to succeed! After each month there will be an opportunity to reflect and reframe your goals and action steps.

Ex. Goal: *Reach my A1C goal of 6.5*

Ex. SMART Action Step: *Use my DHJ at least 5/7 days a week for the next 3 mo.*

Goal #1: _____

1 SMART Action Step: _____

Goal #2: _____

1 SMART Action Step: _____

Goal #3: _____

1 SMART Action Step: _____

1. Why is it important to you to reach these goals? What will you gain from reaching them?

_____

_____

2. What would be the result of not reaching these goals?

_____

_____

> **\*LAUREN'S TIP:** Take an A1C test right before you start the journal, and then schedule one for 3-months out.

# OVERCOMING MY LIMITING BELIEFS

*The beliefs we have about ourselves and the world around us can either be our greatest tool or our most limiting possession. Our beliefs become our reality. Let's choose them wisely.*

Write down three limiting beliefs that you repeatedly tell yourself. These are stories you've constructed in your mind that hold you back you in one way or another. After writing down all three, it's time to let them go. Beneath each, write an empowering statement that in your heart you know is the truth! Let these new beliefs seep into your core over the next three months. See the example below.

**ex.** Disempowering Belief: *High or low blood sugars mean I'm not good enough*

**ex.** New Empowering Belief: *My numbers do not define me. I do my best. I am enough!*

Disempowering Belief: _____

New Empowering Belief: _____

Disempowering Belief: _____

New Empowering Belief: _____

Disempowering Belief: _____

New Empowering Belief: _____

# WRITING MY FUTURE INTO EXISTENCE

*"Although it takes time for these desires to manifest in our material world, you must see the thing you desire as completed, finished, and real, now. The better you can do this, the more you can accomplish."*
*– Terry Crews*

On the lines below, imagine it is three months from now and write a journal entry as if you've already reached your goals. Write down all that you've accomplished, how you feel, and what you did to overcome any roadblocks that came up.

_____

_____

_____

_____

_____

_____

_____

_____

_____

_____

_____

_____

_____

_____

_____

_____

_____

_____

_____

# HOW TO USE THIS JOURNAL

## OVERVIEW

The DHJ contains 90 days of reflection sheets: 7 for each week and a divider separating months one, two, and three. Below is a breakdown of each section of the reflection sheets, and tips for each.

## MORNING WORK IN

Exercising the mind is just as important as exercising the body. In the same way you go to the gym to increase your physical strength, the journal "work in" is meant to increase your mental strength. By preparing your mind each morning, you'll be better ready to conquer whatever daily challenges come your way.

**THE MINDSET PREP HAS 3 PARTS:**

1. **I AM STATEMENT** – Every word we say out loud or to ourselves creates our future. We can speak anything into existence. If you're constantly telling yourself you're not worthy enough, don't have enough time or energy, or aren't capable of making change in your life, your present and future happiness is limited. This space is for you to strengthen your relationship and view of yourself. You can keep this message constant throughout the 3 months or change it day by day depending on what you feel you need.

   **\*LAUREN'S TIP:** Fill out the Morning "Work In" section first thing when you wake up, before looking at your phone or having any human interaction.

2. **Gratitude** – It's easy to focus on what we don't have in our life (and yes, a pancreas that does not fully function makes this list), but thinking about what we DO have allows numerous physiological and physical benefits throughout our day. Gratitude studies show an increase in determination, attention, enthusiasm, and energy, all while improving sleep, lowering anxiety and depression, and making us more resilient against stress. I don't know about you, but I'd like a double shot of that!

   **\*LAUREN'S TIP:** Close your eyes and paint a vivid picture of what you're grateful for. See it, feel it, smile at it. Let that gratitude flood your whole being.

3. **Previous Day Reflection** – This prompt encourages you to look back at the previous day and remind yourself of one thing you didn't do, but that you will do today. Where focus goes, action follows.

## DAILY LOG

These logs are what you'll use throughout the day to track your blood sugar, food, and insulin. You'll start to notice that just with the simple act of writing your blood sugars down you'll start to see improvement in your blood sugars. C/F/P stands for carbs/fat/protein. You don't have to track protein if you don't want to, but I encourage you to become more mindful about the fat content in foods and how it might affect your blood sugar 3-6 hours later. In the note section, be really, really detailed. The more details you have, the more you'll be able to easily identify patterns. Notes can consist of whether you pre-bolused or not, if you were sick that day, if it was your time of the month, if you got little sleep the night before, if you think your pump site is going bad, or if you ate out and the C/F/P were estimated and not exact. I encourage you to test *at least* 5 times a day. And if you have a CGM, make sure to note that it was a CGM reading and not an actual finger prick.

   **\*LAUREN'S TIP:**
   • You can bring your notebook everywhere with you or log numbers in note section of your phone and transfer at night (try to be consistent with whichever method you choose).
   • Saturday and Sunday will be most tempting to skip logging. Aim to log on at least one

weekend day.
- If you feel yourself getting overwhelmed by the logs or if you feel obsessive thoughts, or perfectionistic tendencies coming on, take a break.

## EXERCISE

You can use this space to track/plan your workouts.

 *LAUREN'S TIP: Fill in your exercise slots on Sunday night as a way to plan your week. By taking the decision process out of what you'll do each day for movement, you're more likely to make it happen.

## TOTAL DAILY INSULIN

Record your total daily insulin totals including both fast acting/bolus and long acting/ basal insulin.

## WATER

As you go through the day, shade in the water cups to track your intake. Drinking enough water not only helps prevent high blood sugar, but it also curbs sugar cravings.

 *LAUREN'S TIP:
- If you struggle with remembering to drink water, you can set an alarm on your phone for every 2 hours to alert you, or you can purchase a large water bottle to always keep nearby.
- To figure out how much water you should be drinking, take your body weight in pounds, divide it by 2, and that's how many ounces you should be drinking daily. 8 ounces = 1 cup

## EVENING REFLECTION

The evening reflection page encourages you to set aside time to look back on your day and see how different choices influenced your blood sugars and all around mental and emotional health. You'll ultimately be able to identify what is working for you and what is working against you so you can better prepare yourself for the following day.

*LAUREN'S TIP: Keep a pen by your bedside and fill this section out before bed. Use it as your wind down time.

## HOW I FELT

Take a moment to reflect on how you felt that day and place a check in the corresponding box.

*LAUREN'S TIP: Try not to be judgmental of yourself if you're not "on fire" every single day. You're human, and what matters is that we notice and see how we can improve the next day.

## TODAY I...

For this section, there is a list of mindful habits that elevate the mind, body, and soul. Check off the ones you engage in that day, and use the blank spaces to write any of your own personal joys.

## THE NIGHT CAP

1. **Pattern Recognized** – Look back on your day and find connections between how you felt, the activities you engaged or didn't engage in, and your blood sugars.
2. **Tomorrow's Focus** – Be clear and specific about what you want to focus on the next day.

   *LAUREN'S TIP: Close your eyes and imagine yourself the next day implementing that intentional action step.
3. **Self Celebration** – While it's important to be aware of the areas we can improve upon, get in the habit of celebrating all of your accomplishments, even the smallest ones. When you stop to recognize what accomplishments feel good, you'll prime your mind and body to subconsciously seek out more of those.

# MORNING WORK IN

## MINDSET PREP

I AM... *Energized + ready for a day of progress!*

ONE THING I'M GRATEFUL FOR IS...

*The beautiful colors of this mornings sunrise*

ONE THING I DIDN'T DO YESTERDAY, BUT I WILL DO TODAY...

*Remember to prebolus breakfast as soon as I wake up*

## DAILY LOG

| TIME | BLOOD SUGAR | OUT OF RANGE (x) | INSULIN | C/F/P | NOTES / FOOD |
|---|---|---|---|---|---|
| 7:15am | 110 | | 4.0 | 40c18f15p | ½ cup oats + ½ cup berries |
| 9:32am | 195 | X | 3.2 | 25c3f13p | 2.5 units for pretzels + 0.7 correction |
| 12:32pm | 131 | | 5.2 | 50c20f15p | Shrimp + half avocado wrap (guessed carbs) |
| 2:56pm | 98 | | -- | ----- | Lunch carb guess was right! Mid-day meditation |
| | | | | | |
| | | | | | |
| | | | | | |
| | | | | | |
| | | | | | |
| | | | | | |

# EVENING REFLECTION

Keep an eye out for inspirational quotes, motivating messages, and journal prompts in this section to help you as you go through this process!

| HOW I FELT | 1 (DISSATISFIED) | 2 | 3 (SO-SO) | 4 | 5 (ON FIRE!) |
|---|---|---|---|---|---|
| MOOD | | | | ✓ | |
| ENERGY | | | ✓ | | |
| BLOOD SUGAR | ✓ | | | | |
| NUTRITION | | ✓ | | | |
| MINDSET | | | | | ✓ |

## TODAY I...

- ☑ EXERCISED
- ☐ MEDITATED
- ☑ EXPRESSED GRATITUDE
- ☐ SET GOALS FOR TODAY

- ☑ CHECKED MY SUGAR EVERY 2 HOURS
- ☐ WAS MINDFUL WHEN EATING
- ☐ MEAL PREPPED
- ☑ CARB COUNTED FOOD

- ☑ VISUALIZED DAY OF GOOD BLOOD SUGARS
- ☐ TOOK 10 DEEP BREATHS
- ☑ PRE-BOLUSED MEALS
- ☑ SPENT TIME WITH LOVED ONES

- ☐ TOOK A WALK OUTSIDE
- ☑ *Let go of my anxious thoughts*
- ☑ *Celebrated my in range blood sugars*
- ☐ _____

EXERCISE: *30 minutes on stair master + 20 minutes yoga*

WATER: ▓ ▓ ▓ ▓ ▢ ▢ ▢ ▢ ▢ ▢          TOTAL DAILY INSULIN: *35* UNITS

## THE NIGHT CAP

A PATTERN I RECOGNIZED WAS...

*When I don't eat enough vegetables during the day, I crave more sweets at night*

TOMORROW I WANT TO FOCUS MORE ON...

*Meal prepping my food before going to work*

TODAY I CELEBRATE MYSELF BECAUSE...

*I woke up with an in range number + it set the tone for a good day*

# WEEKLY CHALLENGE LIST

As you dive into the reflection pages, you'll see that at the start of each month, there will be a space to record weekly challenges of your choosing. You may write down all four of your challenges on the first of the month if you'd like, or select them one at a time at the start of each week. These challenges are intended to break you out of your comfort zone and introduce you to new concepts that will elevate your mind, body, and soul. It is up to you which challenges you choose for each week, but do your best to pull from all three categories. Sometimes we gravitate towards what comes easy to us and we resist what is the hardest, but quite often what is hard for us is actually what we need the most. For example, if at first you find yourself choosing only challenges specific to the mind, see if you can be intentional about choosing more body or soul challenges in the following weeks. You may pick your mini challenges from the lists below, or simply come up with any of your own that are calling your name! You are commander in chief of your life. I am your guide, but you're ultimately the one steering the ship.

## MIND

- Eat meals without your phone
- Delete your social media apps
- Read for 20 minutes before bed
- Meditate for 5 minutes each day
- Watch "Hungry for Change" on Netflix
- Listen to a podcast during your commute
- No technology 1 hour before bed
- Sleep with phone on airplane mode
- Listen to a song every morning that puts you in a good mood
- Each morning, visualize what you want your day to look like
- Make a list of 7 things in your life that are not serving you. Write down 1 step you will take each day to let go of each
- Make a list of the challenges in your life and write down why you are GRATEFUL for them
- Each day, un-follow one person on social media whose posts are not serving you

## BODY

- Go caffeine free
- Get 8 hours of sleep
- Eliminate added sugars
- Eat vegetarian or vegan
- Treat yourself to a massage
- Eat 5 servings of vegetables
- Basal/long acting insulin test
- 20 minute walk outside per day
- Commit to [#] of homemade meals
- Finish eating 4 hours before bed time
- Try intermittent fasting for 12-16 hours
- Take a workout class you haven't taken before
- Eliminate gluten and/or dairy to reduce inflammation
- Drink warm lemon water first thing in the morning
- 10 minutes of stretching every morning and/or evening

## SOUL

- Make a new recipe
- Create a vision board
- Watch the sunrise/sunset
- Give 3 compliments per day
- Dance to your favorite music
- De-clutter a room of your home
- Spend time with a family member
- Give people your undivided attention when they're speaking to you
- Have the uncomfortable conversation you've been putting off
- Spend time in nature, sitting with trees or by the water
- Do a random act of kindness every day for a stranger
- Flex your creative muscles and make some type of art

# DEAR SELF, YOU ARE THE GREATEST PROJECT YOU WILL EVER GET TO WORK ON. YOU ARE YOUR OWN HEALER, FRIEND, AND TEACHER.

— LNB

# EVERY JOURNEY BEGINS WITH A SINGLE STEP

# MONTH 01

## WEEKLY CHALLENGE

WEEK 01 _____

_____ ☐ DONE

WEEK 02 _____

_____ ☐ DONE

WEEK 03 _____

_____ ☐ DONE

WEEK 04 _____

_____ ☐ DONE

# MORNING WORK IN | DATE: _____ S / M / T / W / T / F / S

I AM... _____

ONE THING I'M GRATEFUL FOR IS...

_____

ONE THING I DIDN'T DO YESTERDAY, BUT I WILL DO TODAY...

_____

## DAILY LOG

| TIME | BLOOD SUGAR | OUT OF RANGE (x) | INSULIN | C / F / P | NOTES / FOOD |
|------|-------------|------------------|---------|-----------|--------------|
|      |             |                  |         |           |              |
|      |             |                  |         |           |              |
|      |             |                  |         |           |              |
|      |             |                  |         |           |              |
|      |             |                  |         |           |              |
|      |             |                  |         |           |              |
|      |             |                  |         |           |              |
|      |             |                  |         |           |              |
|      |             |                  |         |           |              |
|      |             |                  |         |           |              |

# EVENING REFLECTION

"Progress is not achieved by luck or accident, but by working on yourself daily." – Epictetus

| HOW I FELT | 1 (DISSATISFIED) | 2 | 3 (SO-SO) | 4 | 5 (ON FIRE!) |
|---|---|---|---|---|---|
| MOOD | | | | | |
| ENERGY | | | | | |
| BLOOD SUGAR | | | | | |
| NUTRITION | | | | | |
| MINDSET | | | | | |

## TODAY I...

- [ ] EXERCISED
- [ ] MEDITATED
- [ ] EXPRESSED GRATITUDE
- [ ] SET GOALS FOR TODAY

- [ ] CHECKED MY SUGAR EVERY 2 HOURS
- [ ] WAS MINDFUL WHEN EATING
- [ ] MEAL PREPPED
- [ ] CARB COUNTED FOOD

- [ ] VISUALIZED DAY OF GOOD BLOOD SUGARS
- [ ] TOOK 10 DEEP BREATHS
- [ ] PRE-BOLUSED MEALS
- [ ] SPENT TIME WITH LOVED ONES

- [ ] TOOK A WALK OUTSIDE
- [ ] _____
- [ ] _____
- [ ] _____

EXERCISE: _____

WATER: 🥛 🥛 🥛 🥛 🥛 🥛 🥛 🥛 🥛 🥛          TOTAL DAILY INSULIN: _____ UNITS

## THE NIGHT CAP

A PATTERN I RECOGNIZED WAS...

_____

_____

TOMORROW I WANT TO FOCUS MORE ON...

_____

_____

TODAY I CELEBRATE MYSELF BECAUSE...

_____

_____

# MORNING WORK IN | DATE: _____

## MINDSET PREP

I AM... _____

ONE THING I'M GRATEFUL FOR IS...

_____

ONE THING I DIDN'T DO YESTERDAY, BUT I WILL DO TODAY...

_____

## DAILY LOG

| TIME | BLOOD SUGAR | OUT OF RANGE (x) | INSULIN | C / F / P | NOTES / FOOD |
|------|-------------|------------------|---------|-----------|--------------|
|      |             |                  |         |           |              |
|      |             |                  |         |           |              |
|      |             |                  |         |           |              |
|      |             |                  |         |           |              |
|      |             |                  |         |           |              |
|      |             |                  |         |           |              |
|      |             |                  |         |           |              |
|      |             |                  |         |           |              |
|      |             |                  |         |           |              |

# EVENING REFLECTION | "The mind is just as malleable as the body." – Naval Ravikant

| HOW I FELT | 1 (DISSATISFIED) | 2 | 3 (SO-SO) | 4 | 5 (ON FIRE!) |
|---|---|---|---|---|---|
| MOOD | | | | | |
| ENERGY | | | | | |
| BLOOD SUGAR | | | | | |
| NUTRITION | | | | | |
| MINDSET | | | | | |

## TODAY I...

- ☐ EXERCISED
- ☐ MEDITATED
- ☐ EXPRESSED GRATITUDE
- ☐ SET GOALS FOR TODAY

- ☐ CHECKED MY SUGAR EVERY 2 HOURS
- ☐ WAS MINDFUL WHEN EATING
- ☐ MEAL PREPPED
- ☐ CARB COUNTED FOOD

- ☐ VISUALIZED DAY OF GOOD BLOOD SUGARS
- ☐ TOOK 10 DEEP BREATHS
- ☐ PRE-BOLUSED MEALS
- ☐ SPENT TIME WITH LOVED ONES

- ☐ TOOK A WALK OUTSIDE
- ☐ _____
- ☐ _____
- ☐ _____

EXERCISE: _____

WATER: ☐ ☐ ☐ ☐ ☐ ☐ ☐ ☐ ☐ ☐     TOTAL DAILY INSULIN: _____ UNITS

## THE NIGHT CAP

A PATTERN I RECOGNIZED WAS...

_____

_____

TOMORROW I WANT TO FOCUS MORE ON...

_____

_____

TODAY I CELEBRATE MYSELF BECAUSE...

_____

_____

# MORNING WORK IN

## MINDSET PREP

I AM... _____

ONE THING I'M GRATEFUL FOR IS...

_____

ONE THING I DIDN'T DO YESTERDAY, BUT I WILL DO TODAY...

_____

## DAILY LOG

| TIME | BLOOD SUGAR | OUT OF RANGE (x) | INSULIN | C / F / P | NOTES / FOOD |
|------|-------------|------------------|---------|-----------|--------------|
|      |             |                  |         |           |              |
|      |             |                  |         |           |              |
|      |             |                  |         |           |              |
|      |             |                  |         |           |              |
|      |             |                  |         |           |              |
|      |             |                  |         |           |              |
|      |             |                  |         |           |              |
|      |             |                  |         |           |              |
|      |             |                  |         |           |              |

# EVENING REFLECTION | *Grow through what you go through.*

| HOW I FELT | 1<br>(DISSATISFIED) | 2 | 3<br>(SO-SO) | 4 | 5<br>(ON FIRE!) |
|---|---|---|---|---|---|
| MOOD | | | | | |
| ENERGY | | | | | |
| BLOOD SUGAR | | | | | |
| NUTRITION | | | | | |
| MINDSET | | | | | |

## TODAY I...

☐ EXERCISED

☐ MEDITATED

☐ EXPRESSED GRATITUDE

☐ SET GOALS FOR TODAY

☐ CHECKED MY SUGAR EVERY 2 HOURS

☐ WAS MINDFUL WHEN EATING

☐ MEAL PREPPED

☐ CARB COUNTED FOOD

☐ VISUALIZED DAY OF GOOD BLOOD SUGARS

☐ TOOK 10 DEEP BREATHS

☐ PRE-BOLUSED MEALS

☐ SPENT TIME WITH LOVED ONES

☐ TOOK A WALK OUTSIDE

☐ _____

☐ _____

☐ _____

EXERCISE: _____

WATER: ⊔ ⊔ ⊔ ⊔ ⊔ ⊔ ⊔ ⊔ ⊔ ⊔       TOTAL DAILY INSULIN: _____ UNITS

## THE NIGHT CAP

A PATTERN I RECOGNIZED WAS...

_____

_____

TOMORROW I WANT TO FOCUS MORE ON...

_____

_____

TODAY I CELEBRATE MYSELF BECAUSE...

_____

_____

# MORNING WORK IN | DATE: _____ S / M / T / W / T / F / S

## MINDSET PREP

I AM... _____

ONE THING I'M GRATEFUL FOR IS...

_____

ONE THING I DIDN'T DO YESTERDAY, BUT I WILL DO TODAY...

_____

## DAILY LOG

| TIME | BLOOD SUGAR | OUT OF RANGE (x) | INSULIN | C / F / P | NOTES / FOOD |
|------|-------------|------------------|---------|-----------|--------------|
|      |             |                  |         |           |              |
|      |             |                  |         |           |              |
|      |             |                  |         |           |              |
|      |             |                  |         |           |              |
|      |             |                  |         |           |              |
|      |             |                  |         |           |              |
|      |             |                  |         |           |              |
|      |             |                  |         |           |              |
|      |             |                  |         |           |              |

# EVENING REFLECTION

"When you think you've reached your absolute limit, know that you've only tapped into about 40% of what you're truly capable of." – Rich Roll

## HOW I FELT

| | 1 (DISSATISFIED) | 2 | 3 (SO-SO) | 4 | 5 (ON FIRE!) |
|---|---|---|---|---|---|
| MOOD | | | | | |
| ENERGY | | | | | |
| BLOOD SUGAR | | | | | |
| NUTRITION | | | | | |
| MINDSET | | | | | |

## TODAY I...

- ☐ EXERCISED
- ☐ CHECKED MY SUGAR EVERY 2 HOURS
- ☐ VISUALIZED DAY OF GOOD BLOOD SUGARS
- ☐ TOOK A WALK OUTSIDE

- ☐ MEDITATED
- ☐ WAS MINDFUL WHEN EATING
- ☐ TOOK 10 DEEP BREATHS
- ☐ _____

- ☐ EXPRESSED GRATITUDE
- ☐ MEAL PREPPED
- ☐ PRE-BOLUSED MEALS
- ☐ _____

- ☐ SET GOALS FOR TODAY
- ☐ CARB COUNTED FOOD
- ☐ SPENT TIME WITH LOVED ONES
- ☐ _____

EXERCISE: _____

WATER: ☐ ☐ ☐ ☐ ☐ ☐ ☐ ☐ ☐ ☐     TOTAL DAILY INSULIN: _____ UNITS

## THE NIGHT CAP

A PATTERN I RECOGNIZED WAS...

_____

_____

TOMORROW I WANT TO FOCUS MORE ON...

_____

_____

TODAY I CELEBRATE MYSELF BECAUSE...

_____

_____

# MORNING WORK IN | DATE: _____ S / M / T / W / T / F / S

## MINDSET PREP

I AM... _____

ONE THING I'M GRATEFUL FOR IS...

_____

ONE THING I DIDN'T DO YESTERDAY, BUT I WILL DO TODAY...

_____

## DAILY LOG

| TIME | BLOOD SUGAR | OUT OF RANGE (x) | INSULIN | C / F / P | NOTES / FOOD |
|------|-------------|------------------|---------|-----------|--------------|
|      |             |                  |         |           |              |
|      |             |                  |         |           |              |
|      |             |                  |         |           |              |
|      |             |                  |         |           |              |
|      |             |                  |         |           |              |
|      |             |                  |         |           |              |
|      |             |                  |         |           |              |
|      |             |                  |         |           |              |
|      |             |                  |         |           |              |

# EVENING REFLECTION

"I am convinced that life is 10% what happens to me and 90% of how I react to it." – Charles R. Swindoll

| HOW I FELT | 1 (DISSATISFIED) | 2 | 3 (SO-SO) | 4 | 5 (ON FIRE!) |
|---|---|---|---|---|---|
| MOOD | | | | | |
| ENERGY | | | | | |
| BLOOD SUGAR | | | | | |
| NUTRITION | | | | | |
| MINDSET | | | | | |

## TODAY I...

- ☐ EXERCISED
- ☐ MEDITATED
- ☐ EXPRESSED GRATITUDE
- ☐ SET GOALS FOR TODAY

- ☐ CHECKED MY SUGAR EVERY 2 HOURS
- ☐ WAS MINDFUL WHEN EATING
- ☐ MEAL PREPPED
- ☐ CARB COUNTED FOOD

- ☐ VISUALIZED DAY OF GOOD BLOOD SUGARS
- ☐ TOOK 10 DEEP BREATHS
- ☐ PRE-BOLUSED MEALS
- ☐ SPENT TIME WITH LOVED ONES

- ☐ TOOK A WALK OUTSIDE
- ☐ _____
- ☐ _____
- ☐ _____

EXERCISE: _____

WATER: ⊔ ⊔ ⊔ ⊔ ⊔ ⊔ ⊔ ⊔ ⊔ ⊔    TOTAL DAILY INSULIN: _____ UNITS

## THE NIGHT CAP

A PATTERN I RECOGNIZED WAS...

_____

_____

TOMORROW I WANT TO FOCUS MORE ON...

_____

_____

TODAY I CELEBRATE MYSELF BECAUSE...

_____

_____

# MORNING WORK IN | DATE: _____ S / M / T / W / T / F / S

## MINDSET PREP          I AM... _____

ONE THING I'M GRATEFUL FOR IS...

_____

ONE THING I DIDN'T DO YESTERDAY, BUT I WILL DO TODAY...

_____

## DAILY LOG

| TIME | BLOOD SUGAR | OUT OF RANGE (x) | INSULIN | C / F / P | NOTES / FOOD |
|------|-------------|------------------|---------|-----------|--------------|
|      |             |                  |         |           |              |
|      |             |                  |         |           |              |
|      |             |                  |         |           |              |
|      |             |                  |         |           |              |
|      |             |                  |         |           |              |
|      |             |                  |         |           |              |
|      |             |                  |         |           |              |
|      |             |                  |         |           |              |
|      |             |                  |         |           |              |

# EVENING REFLECTION

**JOURNAL PROMPT:**
What would happen today if you based all of your decisions on what would give you the most energy?

| HOW I FELT | 1 (DISSATISFIED) | 2 | 3 (SO-SO) | 4 | 5 (ON FIRE!) |
|---|---|---|---|---|---|
| MOOD | | | | | |
| ENERGY | | | | | |
| BLOOD SUGAR | | | | | |
| NUTRITION | | | | | |
| MINDSET | | | | | |

## TODAY I...

☐ EXERCISED    ☐ CHECKED MY SUGAR EVERY 2 HOURS    ☐ VISUALIZED DAY OF GOOD BLOOD SUGARS    ☐ TOOK A WALK OUTSIDE

☐ MEDITATED    ☐ WAS MINDFUL WHEN EATING    ☐ TOOK 10 DEEP BREATHS    ☐ _____

☐ EXPRESSED GRATITUDE    ☐ MEAL PREPPED    ☐ PRE-BOLUSED MEALS    ☐ _____

☐ SET GOALS FOR TODAY    ☐ CARB COUNTED FOOD    ☐ SPENT TIME WITH LOVED ONES    ☐ _____

EXERCISE: _____

WATER: ☐ ☐ ☐ ☐ ☐ ☐ ☐ ☐ ☐ ☐     TOTAL DAILY INSULIN: _____ UNITS

## THE NIGHT CAP

A PATTERN I RECOGNIZED WAS...

_____

_____

TOMORROW I WANT TO FOCUS MORE ON...

_____

_____

TODAY I CELEBRATE MYSELF BECAUSE...

_____

_____

# MORNING WORK IN | DATE: _____ S / M / T / W / T / F / S

## MINDSET PREP

I AM... _____

ONE THING I'M GRATEFUL FOR IS...

_____

ONE THING I DIDN'T DO YESTERDAY, BUT I WILL DO TODAY...

_____

## DAILY LOG

| TIME | BLOOD SUGAR | OUT OF RANGE (x) | INSULIN | C / F / P | NOTES / FOOD |
|------|-------------|------------------|---------|-----------|--------------|
|      |             |                  |         |           |              |
|      |             |                  |         |           |              |
|      |             |                  |         |           |              |
|      |             |                  |         |           |              |
|      |             |                  |         |           |              |
|      |             |                  |         |           |              |
|      |             |                  |         |           |              |
|      |             |                  |         |           |              |
|      |             |                  |         |           |              |
|      |             |                  |         |           |              |

# EVENING REFLECTION

"How you love yourself is how you teach others to love you."
– Rupi Kaur

## HOW I FELT

| | 1 (DISSATISFIED) | 2 | 3 (SO-SO) | 4 | 5 (ON FIRE!) |
|---|---|---|---|---|---|
| MOOD | | | | | |
| ENERGY | | | | | |
| BLOOD SUGAR | | | | | |
| NUTRITION | | | | | |
| MINDSET | | | | | |

## TODAY I...

☐ EXERCISED

☐ MEDITATED

☐ EXPRESSED GRATITUDE

☐ SET GOALS FOR TODAY

☐ CHECKED MY SUGAR EVERY 2 HOURS

☐ WAS MINDFUL WHEN EATING

☐ MEAL PREPPED

☐ CARB COUNTED FOOD

☐ VISUALIZED DAY OF GOOD BLOOD SUGARS

☐ TOOK 10 DEEP BREATHS

☐ PRE-BOLUSED MEALS

☐ SPENT TIME WITH LOVED ONES

☐ TOOK A WALK OUTSIDE

☐ _____

☐ _____

☐ _____

EXERCISE: _____

WATER: ☐ ☐ ☐ ☐ ☐ ☐ ☐ ☐ ☐ ☐          TOTAL DAILY INSULIN: _____ UNITS

## THE NIGHT CAP

A PATTERN I RECOGNIZED WAS...

_____

_____

TOMORROW I WANT TO FOCUS MORE ON...

_____

_____

TODAY I CELEBRATE MYSELF BECAUSE...

_____

_____

# MORNING WORK IN | DATE: _____ S / M / T / W / T / F / S

## MINDSET PREP

I AM... _____

ONE THING I'M GRATEFUL FOR IS...

_____

ONE THING I DIDN'T DO YESTERDAY, BUT I WILL DO TODAY...

_____

## DAILY LOG

| TIME | BLOOD SUGAR | OUT OF RANGE (x) | INSULIN | C / F / P | NOTES / FOOD |
|------|------|------|------|------|------|
|  |  |  |  |  |  |
|  |  |  |  |  |  |
|  |  |  |  |  |  |
|  |  |  |  |  |  |
|  |  |  |  |  |  |
|  |  |  |  |  |  |
|  |  |  |  |  |  |
|  |  |  |  |  |  |
|  |  |  |  |  |  |

# EVENING REFLECTION

"Do not lower your goals to the level of your abilities. Instead, raise your abilities to the height of your goals."
– Swami Vivekananda

| HOW I FELT | 1 (DISSATISFIED) | 2 | 3 (SO-SO) | 4 | 5 (ON FIRE!) |
|---|---|---|---|---|---|
| MOOD | | | | | |
| ENERGY | | | | | |
| BLOOD SUGAR | | | | | |
| NUTRITION | | | | | |
| MINDSET | | | | | |

## TODAY I...

☐ EXERCISED    ☐ CHECKED MY SUGAR EVERY 2 HOURS    ☐ VISUALIZED DAY OF GOOD BLOOD SUGARS    ☐ TOOK A WALK OUTSIDE

☐ MEDITATED    ☐ WAS MINDFUL WHEN EATING    ☐ TOOK 10 DEEP BREATHS    ☐ _____

☐ EXPRESSED GRATITUDE    ☐ MEAL PREPPED    ☐ PRE-BOLUSED MEALS    ☐ _____

☐ SET GOALS FOR TODAY    ☐ CARB COUNTED FOOD    ☐ SPENT TIME WITH LOVED ONES    ☐ _____

EXERCISE: _____

WATER: ▢ ▢ ▢ ▢ ▢ ▢ ▢ ▢ ▢ ▢    TOTAL DAILY INSULIN: _____ UNITS

## THE NIGHT CAP

A PATTERN I RECOGNIZED WAS...

_____

_____

TOMORROW I WANT TO FOCUS MORE ON...

_____

_____

TODAY I CELEBRATE MYSELF BECAUSE...

_____

_____

# MORNING WORK IN | DATE: _____ S / M / T / W / T / F / S

## MINDSET PREP

I AM... _____

ONE THING I'M GRATEFUL FOR IS...

_____

ONE THING I DIDN'T DO YESTERDAY, BUT I WILL DO TODAY...

_____

## DAILY LOG

| TIME | BLOOD SUGAR | OUT OF RANGE (x) | INSULIN | C / F / P | NOTES / FOOD |
|------|-------------|------------------|---------|-----------|--------------|
|      |             |                  |         |           |              |
|      |             |                  |         |           |              |
|      |             |                  |         |           |              |
|      |             |                  |         |           |              |
|      |             |                  |         |           |              |
|      |             |                  |         |           |              |
|      |             |                  |         |           |              |
|      |             |                  |         |           |              |
|      |             |                  |         |           |              |
|      |             |                  |         |           |              |

# EVENING REFLECTION | "It is the power of the mind to be unconquerable." – Seneca

| HOW I FELT | 1 (DISSATISFIED) | 2 | 3 (SO-SO) | 4 | 5 (ON FIRE!) |
|---|---|---|---|---|---|
| MOOD | | | | | |
| ENERGY | | | | | |
| BLOOD SUGAR | | | | | |
| NUTRITION | | | | | |
| MINDSET | | | | | |

## TODAY I...

- ☐ EXERCISED
- ☐ MEDITATED
- ☐ EXPRESSED GRATITUDE
- ☐ SET GOALS FOR TODAY

- ☐ CHECKED MY SUGAR EVERY 2 HOURS
- ☐ WAS MINDFUL WHEN EATING
- ☐ MEAL PREPPED
- ☐ CARB COUNTED FOOD

- ☐ VISUALIZED DAY OF GOOD BLOOD SUGARS
- ☐ TOOK 10 DEEP BREATHS
- ☐ PRE-BOLUSED MEALS
- ☐ SPENT TIME WITH LOVED ONES

- ☐ TOOK A WALK OUTSIDE
- ☐ _____
- ☐ _____
- ☐ _____

EXERCISE: _____

WATER: ▯ ▯ ▯ ▯ ▯ ▯ ▯ ▯ ▯ ▯    TOTAL DAILY INSULIN: _____ UNITS

## THE NIGHT CAP

A PATTERN I RECOGNIZED WAS...

_____

_____

TOMORROW I WANT TO FOCUS MORE ON...

_____

_____

TODAY I CELEBRATE MYSELF BECAUSE...

_____

_____

# MORNING WORK IN | DATE: _____ S / M / T / W / T / F / S

## MINDSET PREP

I AM... _____

ONE THING I'M GRATEFUL FOR IS...

_____

ONE THING I DIDN'T DO YESTERDAY, BUT I WILL DO TODAY...

_____

## DAILY LOG

| TIME | BLOOD SUGAR | OUT OF RANGE (x) | INSULIN | C / F / P | NOTES / FOOD |
|------|-------------|------------------|---------|-----------|--------------|
|      |             |                  |         |           |              |
|      |             |                  |         |           |              |
|      |             |                  |         |           |              |
|      |             |                  |         |           |              |
|      |             |                  |         |           |              |
|      |             |                  |         |           |              |
|      |             |                  |         |           |              |
|      |             |                  |         |           |              |
|      |             |                  |         |           |              |
|      |             |                  |         |           |              |

# EVENING REFLECTION | *Aim for progress, not perfection.*

| HOW I FELT | 1 (DISSATISFIED) | 2 | 3 (SO-SO) | 4 | 5 (ON FIRE!) |
|---|---|---|---|---|---|
| MOOD | | | | | |
| ENERGY | | | | | |
| BLOOD SUGAR | | | | | |
| NUTRITION | | | | | |
| MINDSET | | | | | |

## TODAY I...

- ☐ EXERCISED
- ☐ MEDITATED
- ☐ EXPRESSED GRATITUDE
- ☐ SET GOALS FOR TODAY

- ☐ CHECKED MY SUGAR EVERY 2 HOURS
- ☐ WAS MINDFUL WHEN EATING
- ☐ MEAL PREPPED
- ☐ CARB COUNTED FOOD

- ☐ VISUALIZED DAY OF GOOD BLOOD SUGARS
- ☐ TOOK 10 DEEP BREATHS
- ☐ PRE-BOLUSED MEALS
- ☐ SPENT TIME WITH LOVED ONES

- ☐ TOOK A WALK OUTSIDE
- ☐ _____
- ☐ _____
- ☐ _____

EXERCISE: _____

WATER: ☐ ☐ ☐ ☐ ☐ ☐ ☐ ☐ ☐ ☐     TOTAL DAILY INSULIN: _____ UNITS

## THE NIGHT CAP

A PATTERN I RECOGNIZED WAS...

_____

_____

TOMORROW I WANT TO FOCUS MORE ON...

_____

_____

TODAY I CELEBRATE MYSELF BECAUSE...

_____

_____

# MORNING WORK IN | DATE: _____ S / M / T / W / T / F / S

## MINDSET PREP

I AM... _____

ONE THING I'M GRATEFUL FOR IS...

_____

ONE THING I DIDN'T DO YESTERDAY, BUT I WILL DO TODAY...

_____

## DAILY LOG

| TIME | BLOOD SUGAR | OUT OF RANGE (x) | INSULIN | C / F / P | NOTES / FOOD |
|------|-------------|------------------|---------|-----------|--------------|
|      |             |                  |         |           |              |
|      |             |                  |         |           |              |
|      |             |                  |         |           |              |
|      |             |                  |         |           |              |
|      |             |                  |         |           |              |
|      |             |                  |         |           |              |
|      |             |                  |         |           |              |
|      |             |                  |         |           |              |
|      |             |                  |         |           |              |
|      |             |                  |         |           |              |

# EVENING REFLECTION | "Don't let yesterday take up too much of today." – Will Rogers

| HOW I FELT | 1 (DISSATISFIED) | 2 | 3 (SO-SO) | 4 | 5 (ON FIRE!) |
|---|---|---|---|---|---|
| MOOD | | | | | |
| ENERGY | | | | | |
| BLOOD SUGAR | | | | | |
| NUTRITION | | | | | |
| MINDSET | | | | | |

## TODAY I...

- ☐ EXERCISED
- ☐ CHECKED MY SUGAR EVERY 2 HOURS
- ☐ VISUALIZED DAY OF GOOD BLOOD SUGARS
- ☐ TOOK A WALK OUTSIDE

- ☐ MEDITATED
- ☐ WAS MINDFUL WHEN EATING
- ☐ TOOK 10 DEEP BREATHS
- ☐ _____

- ☐ EXPRESSED GRATITUDE
- ☐ MEAL PREPPED
- ☐ PRE-BOLUSED MEALS
- ☐ _____

- ☐ SET GOALS FOR TODAY
- ☐ CARB COUNTED FOOD
- ☐ SPENT TIME WITH LOVED ONES
- ☐ _____

EXERCISE: _____

WATER: ☐ ☐ ☐ ☐ ☐ ☐ ☐ ☐ ☐ ☐          TOTAL DAILY INSULIN: _____ UNITS

## THE NIGHT CAP

A PATTERN I RECOGNIZED WAS...

_____

_____

TOMORROW I WANT TO FOCUS MORE ON...

_____

_____

TODAY I CELEBRATE MYSELF BECAUSE...

_____

_____

# MORNING WORK IN

DATE: _____ S / M / T / W / T / F / S

## MINDSET PREP

I AM... _____

ONE THING I'M GRATEFUL FOR IS...

_____

ONE THING I DIDN'T DO YESTERDAY, BUT I WILL DO TODAY...

_____

## DAILY LOG

| TIME | BLOOD SUGAR | OUT OF RANGE (x) | INSULIN | C / F / P | NOTES / FOOD |
|------|-------------|------------------|---------|-----------|--------------|
|      |             |                  |         |           |              |
|      |             |                  |         |           |              |
|      |             |                  |         |           |              |
|      |             |                  |         |           |              |
|      |             |                  |         |           |              |
|      |             |                  |         |           |              |
|      |             |                  |         |           |              |
|      |             |                  |         |           |              |
|      |             |                  |         |           |              |
|      |             |                  |         |           |              |

# EVENING REFLECTION | JOURNAL PROMPT:
What is one thing you are looking forward to today?

| HOW I FELT | 1 (DISSATISFIED) | 2 | 3 (SO-SO) | 4 | 5 (ON FIRE!) |
|---|---|---|---|---|---|
| MOOD | | | | | |
| ENERGY | | | | | |
| BLOOD SUGAR | | | | | |
| NUTRITION | | | | | |
| MINDSET | | | | | |

## TODAY I...

☐ EXERCISED      ☐ CHECKED MY SUGAR      ☐ VISUALIZED DAY OF      ☐ TOOK A WALK OUTSIDE
                     EVERY 2 HOURS             GOOD BLOOD SUGARS

☐ MEDITATED      ☐ WAS MINDFUL          ☐ TOOK 10 DEEP          ☐ _____
                     WHEN EATING               BREATHS

☐ EXPRESSED      ☐ MEAL PREPPED         ☐ PRE-BOLUSED           ☐ _____
   GRATITUDE                                  MEALS

☐ SET GOALS      ☐ CARB COUNTED         ☐ SPENT TIME WITH       ☐ _____
   FOR TODAY          FOOD                     LOVED ONES

EXERCISE: _____

WATER: ▯ ▯ ▯ ▯ ▯ ▯ ▯ ▯ ▯ ▯     TOTAL DAILY INSULIN: _____ UNITS

## THE NIGHT CAP

A PATTERN I RECOGNIZED WAS...

_____

_____

TOMORROW I WANT TO FOCUS MORE ON...

_____

_____

TODAY I CELEBRATE MYSELF BECAUSE...

_____

_____

# MORNING WORK IN | DATE: _____ S / M / T / W / T / F / S

## MINDSET PREP

I AM... _____

ONE THING I'M GRATEFUL FOR IS...

_____

ONE THING I DIDN'T DO YESTERDAY, BUT I WILL DO TODAY...

_____

## DAILY LOG

| TIME | BLOOD SUGAR | OUT OF RANGE (x) | INSULIN | C / F / P | NOTES / FOOD |
|------|-------------|------------------|---------|-----------|--------------|
|      |             |                  |         |           |              |
|      |             |                  |         |           |              |
|      |             |                  |         |           |              |
|      |             |                  |         |           |              |
|      |             |                  |         |           |              |
|      |             |                  |         |           |              |
|      |             |                  |         |           |              |
|      |             |                  |         |           |              |
|      |             |                  |         |           |              |
|      |             |                  |         |           |              |

# EVENING REFLECTION

"You don't need to prove to others you are good enough if you believe it yourself." – LNB

| HOW I FELT | 1 (DISSATISFIED) | 2 | 3 (SO-SO) | 4 | 5 (ON FIRE!) |
|---|---|---|---|---|---|
| MOOD | | | | | |
| ENERGY | | | | | |
| BLOOD SUGAR | | | | | |
| NUTRITION | | | | | |
| MINDSET | | | | | |

## TODAY I...

- ☐ EXERCISED
- ☐ MEDITATED
- ☐ EXPRESSED GRATITUDE
- ☐ SET GOALS FOR TODAY

- ☐ CHECKED MY SUGAR EVERY 2 HOURS
- ☐ WAS MINDFUL WHEN EATING
- ☐ MEAL PREPPED
- ☐ CARB COUNTED FOOD

- ☐ VISUALIZED DAY OF GOOD BLOOD SUGARS
- ☐ TOOK 10 DEEP BREATHS
- ☐ PRE-BOLUSED MEALS
- ☐ SPENT TIME WITH LOVED ONES

- ☐ TOOK A WALK OUTSIDE
- ☐ _____
- ☐ _____
- ☐ _____

EXERCISE: _____

WATER: ▽ ▽ ▽ ▽ ▽ ▽ ▽ ▽ ▽ ▽          TOTAL DAILY INSULIN: _____ UNITS

## THE NIGHT CAP

A PATTERN I RECOGNIZED WAS...

_____

_____

TOMORROW I WANT TO FOCUS MORE ON...

_____

_____

TODAY I CELEBRATE MYSELF BECAUSE...

_____

_____

# MORNING WORK IN | DATE: _____ S / M / T / W / T / F / S

## MINDSET PREP

I AM... _____

ONE THING I'M GRATEFUL FOR IS...

_____

ONE THING I DIDN'T DO YESTERDAY, BUT I WILL DO TODAY...

_____

## DAILY LOG

| TIME | BLOOD SUGAR | OUT OF RANGE (x) | INSULIN | C / F / P | NOTES / FOOD |
|------|-------------|------------------|---------|-----------|--------------|
|      |             |                  |         |           |              |
|      |             |                  |         |           |              |
|      |             |                  |         |           |              |
|      |             |                  |         |           |              |
|      |             |                  |         |           |              |
|      |             |                  |         |           |              |
|      |             |                  |         |           |              |
|      |             |                  |         |           |              |
|      |             |                  |         |           |              |

# EVENING REFLECTION
"If you have the ability to love, love yourself first."
– Charles Bukowski

| HOW I FELT | 1 (DISSATISFIED) | 2 | 3 (SO-SO) | 4 | 5 (ON FIRE!) |
|---|---|---|---|---|---|
| MOOD | | | | | |
| ENERGY | | | | | |
| BLOOD SUGAR | | | | | |
| NUTRITION | | | | | |
| MINDSET | | | | | |

## TODAY I...

- ☐ EXERCISED
- ☐ MEDITATED
- ☐ EXPRESSED GRATITUDE
- ☐ SET GOALS FOR TODAY

- ☐ CHECKED MY SUGAR EVERY 2 HOURS
- ☐ WAS MINDFUL WHEN EATING
- ☐ MEAL PREPPED
- ☐ CARB COUNTED FOOD

- ☐ VISUALIZED DAY OF GOOD BLOOD SUGARS
- ☐ TOOK 10 DEEP BREATHS
- ☐ PRE-BOLUSED MEALS
- ☐ SPENT TIME WITH LOVED ONES

- ☐ TOOK A WALK OUTSIDE
- ☐ _____
- ☐ _____
- ☐ _____

EXERCISE: _____

WATER: ☐ ☐ ☐ ☐ ☐ ☐ ☐ ☐ ☐ ☐     TOTAL DAILY INSULIN: _____ UNITS

## THE NIGHT CAP

A PATTERN I RECOGNIZED WAS...

_____

_____

TOMORROW I WANT TO FOCUS MORE ON...

_____

_____

TODAY I CELEBRATE MYSELF BECAUSE...

_____

_____

# MORNING WORK IN | DATE: _____

## MINDSET PREP

I AM... _____

ONE THING I'M GRATEFUL FOR IS...

_____

ONE THING I DIDN'T DO YESTERDAY, BUT I WILL DO TODAY...

_____

## DAILY LOG

| TIME | BLOOD SUGAR | OUT OF RANGE (x) | INSULIN | C / F / P | NOTES / FOOD |
|------|-------------|------------------|---------|-----------|--------------|
|      |             |                  |         |           |              |
|      |             |                  |         |           |              |
|      |             |                  |         |           |              |
|      |             |                  |         |           |              |
|      |             |                  |         |           |              |
|      |             |                  |         |           |              |
|      |             |                  |         |           |              |
|      |             |                  |         |           |              |
|      |             |                  |         |           |              |
|      |             |                  |         |           |              |

# EVENING REFLECTION | "You just can't beat a person who never gives up." – Babe Ruth

| HOW I FELT | 1 (DISSATISFIED) | 2 | 3 (SO-SO) | 4 | 5 (ON FIRE!) |
|---|---|---|---|---|---|
| MOOD | | | | | |
| ENERGY | | | | | |
| BLOOD SUGAR | | | | | |
| NUTRITION | | | | | |
| MINDSET | | | | | |

## TODAY I...

☐ EXERCISED

☐ CHECKED MY SUGAR EVERY 2 HOURS

☐ VISUALIZED DAY OF GOOD BLOOD SUGARS

☐ TOOK A WALK OUTSIDE

☐ MEDITATED

☐ WAS MINDFUL WHEN EATING

☐ TOOK 10 DEEP BREATHS

☐ _____

☐ EXPRESSED GRATITUDE

☐ MEAL PREPPED

☐ PRE-BOLUSED MEALS

☐ _____

☐ SET GOALS FOR TODAY

☐ CARB COUNTED FOOD

☐ SPENT TIME WITH LOVED ONES

☐ _____

EXERCISE: _____

WATER: ▭ ▭ ▭ ▭ ▭ ▭ ▭ ▭ ▭ ▭     TOTAL DAILY INSULIN: _____ UNITS

## THE NIGHT CAP

A PATTERN I RECOGNIZED WAS...

_____

_____

TOMORROW I WANT TO FOCUS MORE ON...

_____

_____

TODAY I CELEBRATE MYSELF BECAUSE...

_____

_____

# MORNING WORK IN | DATE: _____ S / M / T / W / T / F / S

I AM... _____

ONE THING I'M GRATEFUL FOR IS...

_____

ONE THING I DIDN'T DO YESTERDAY, BUT I WILL DO TODAY...

_____

## DAILY LOG

| TIME | BLOOD SUGAR | OUT OF RANGE (x) | INSULIN | C / F / P | NOTES / FOOD |
|------|-------------|------------------|---------|-----------|--------------|
|      |             |                  |         |           |              |
|      |             |                  |         |           |              |
|      |             |                  |         |           |              |
|      |             |                  |         |           |              |
|      |             |                  |         |           |              |
|      |             |                  |         |           |              |
|      |             |                  |         |           |              |
|      |             |                  |         |           |              |
|      |             |                  |         |           |              |
|      |             |                  |         |           |              |

# EVENING REFLECTION | "Difficulties strengthen the mind, as labor does the body."
– Lucius Annaeus Seneca

| HOW I FELT | 1 (DISSATISFIED) | 2 | 3 (SO-SO) | 4 | 5 (ON FIRE!) |
|---|---|---|---|---|---|
| MOOD | | | | | |
| ENERGY | | | | | |
| BLOOD SUGAR | | | | | |
| NUTRITION | | | | | |
| MINDSET | | | | | |

## TODAY I...

- [ ] EXERCISED
- [ ] MEDITATED
- [ ] EXPRESSED GRATITUDE
- [ ] SET GOALS FOR TODAY

- [ ] CHECKED MY SUGAR EVERY 2 HOURS
- [ ] WAS MINDFUL WHEN EATING
- [ ] MEAL PREPPED
- [ ] CARB COUNTED FOOD

- [ ] VISUALIZED DAY OF GOOD BLOOD SUGARS
- [ ] TOOK 10 DEEP BREATHS
- [ ] PRE-BOLUSED MEALS
- [ ] SPENT TIME WITH LOVED ONES

- [ ] TOOK A WALK OUTSIDE
- [ ] _____
- [ ] _____
- [ ] _____

EXERCISE: _____

WATER: ⬜ ⬜ ⬜ ⬜ ⬜ ⬜ ⬜ ⬜ ⬜ ⬜     TOTAL DAILY INSULIN: _____ UNITS

## THE NIGHT CAP

A PATTERN I RECOGNIZED WAS...

_____

_____

TOMORROW I WANT TO FOCUS MORE ON...

_____

_____

TODAY I CELEBRATE MYSELF BECAUSE...

_____

_____

# MORNING WORK IN | DATE: _____ S / M / T / W / T / F / S

## MINDSET PREP

I AM... _____

ONE THING I'M GRATEFUL FOR IS...

_____

ONE THING I DIDN'T DO YESTERDAY, BUT I WILL DO TODAY...

_____

## DAILY LOG

| TIME | BLOOD SUGAR | OUT OF RANGE (x) | INSULIN | C / F / P | NOTES / FOOD |
|------|-------------|------------------|---------|-----------|--------------|
|      |             |                  |         |           |              |
|      |             |                  |         |           |              |
|      |             |                  |         |           |              |
|      |             |                  |         |           |              |
|      |             |                  |         |           |              |
|      |             |                  |         |           |              |
|      |             |                  |         |           |              |
|      |             |                  |         |           |              |
|      |             |                  |         |           |              |

# EVENING REFLECTION | *Don't rush something you want to live forever.*

| HOW I FELT | 1<br>(DISSATISFIED) | 2 | 3<br>(SO-SO) | 4 | 5<br>(ON FIRE!) |
|---|---|---|---|---|---|
| MOOD | | | | | |
| ENERGY | | | | | |
| BLOOD SUGAR | | | | | |
| NUTRITION | | | | | |
| MINDSET | | | | | |

## TODAY I...

- [ ] EXERCISED
- [ ] MEDITATED
- [ ] EXPRESSED GRATITUDE
- [ ] SET GOALS FOR TODAY

- [ ] CHECKED MY SUGAR EVERY 2 HOURS
- [ ] WAS MINDFUL WHEN EATING
- [ ] MEAL PREPPED
- [ ] CARB COUNTED FOOD

- [ ] VISUALIZED DAY OF GOOD BLOOD SUGARS
- [ ] TOOK 10 DEEP BREATHS
- [ ] PRE-BOLUSED MEALS
- [ ] SPENT TIME WITH LOVED ONES

- [ ] TOOK A WALK OUTSIDE
- [ ] _____
- [ ] _____
- [ ] _____

EXERCISE: _____

WATER: ▯ ▯ ▯ ▯ ▯ ▯ ▯ ▯ ▯ ▯      TOTAL DAILY INSULIN: _____ UNITS

## THE NIGHT CAP

A PATTERN I RECOGNIZED WAS...

_____

_____

TOMORROW I WANT TO FOCUS MORE ON...

_____

_____

TODAY I CELEBRATE MYSELF BECAUSE...

_____

_____

# MORNING WORK IN | DATE: _____ S / M / T / W / T / F / S

## MINDSET PREP

I AM... _____

ONE THING I'M GRATEFUL FOR IS...

_____

ONE THING I DIDN'T DO YESTERDAY, BUT I WILL DO TODAY...

_____

## DAILY LOG

| TIME | BLOOD SUGAR | OUT OF RANGE (x) | INSULIN | C / F / P | NOTES / FOOD |
|------|-------------|------------------|---------|-----------|--------------|
|      |             |                  |         |           |              |
|      |             |                  |         |           |              |
|      |             |                  |         |           |              |
|      |             |                  |         |           |              |
|      |             |                  |         |           |              |
|      |             |                  |         |           |              |
|      |             |                  |         |           |              |
|      |             |                  |         |           |              |
|      |             |                  |         |           |              |
|      |             |                  |         |           |              |

# EVENING REFLECTION | "Great things never came from comfort zones." – Ben Francia

| HOW I FELT | 1<br>(DISSATISFIED) | 2 | 3<br>(SO-SO) | 4 | 5<br>(ON FIRE!) |
|---|---|---|---|---|---|
| MOOD | | | | | |
| ENERGY | | | | | |
| BLOOD SUGAR | | | | | |
| NUTRITION | | | | | |
| MINDSET | | | | | |

## TODAY I...

- ☐ EXERCISED
- ☐ MEDITATED
- ☐ EXPRESSED GRATITUDE
- ☐ SET GOALS FOR TODAY

- ☐ CHECKED MY SUGAR EVERY 2 HOURS
- ☐ WAS MINDFUL WHEN EATING
- ☐ MEAL PREPPED
- ☐ CARB COUNTED FOOD

- ☐ VISUALIZED DAY OF GOOD BLOOD SUGARS
- ☐ TOOK 10 DEEP BREATHS
- ☐ PRE-BOLUSED MEALS
- ☐ SPENT TIME WITH LOVED ONES

- ☐ TOOK A WALK OUTSIDE
- ☐ _____
- ☐ _____
- ☐ _____

EXERCISE: _____

WATER: ▽ ▽ ▽ ▽ ▽ ▽ ▽ ▽ ▽ ▽      TOTAL DAILY INSULIN: _____ UNITS

## THE NIGHT CAP

A PATTERN I RECOGNIZED WAS...

_____
_____

TOMORROW I WANT TO FOCUS MORE ON...

_____
_____

TODAY I CELEBRATE MYSELF BECAUSE...

_____
_____

# MORNING WORK IN | DATE: _____ S / M / T / W / T / F / S

## MINDSET PREP | I AM... _____

ONE THING I'M GRATEFUL FOR IS...

_____

ONE THING I DIDN'T DO YESTERDAY, BUT I WILL DO TODAY...

_____

## DAILY LOG

| TIME | BLOOD SUGAR | OUT OF RANGE (x) | INSULIN | C / F / P | NOTES / FOOD |
|------|-------------|------------------|---------|-----------|--------------|
|      |             |                  |         |           |              |
|      |             |                  |         |           |              |
|      |             |                  |         |           |              |
|      |             |                  |         |           |              |
|      |             |                  |         |           |              |
|      |             |                  |         |           |              |
|      |             |                  |         |           |              |
|      |             |                  |         |           |              |
|      |             |                  |         |           |              |
|      |             |                  |         |           |              |

# EVENING REFLECTION | JOURNAL PROMPT:
If you were the bravest version of yourself today, what is one thing you would do?

| HOW I FELT | 1<br>(DISSATISFIED) | 2 | 3<br>(SO-SO) | 4 | 5<br>(ON FIRE!) |
|---|---|---|---|---|---|
| MOOD | | | | | |
| ENERGY | | | | | |
| BLOOD SUGAR | | | | | |
| NUTRITION | | | | | |
| MINDSET | | | | | |

## TODAY I...

- ☐ EXERCISED
- ☐ MEDITATED
- ☐ EXPRESSED GRATITUDE
- ☐ SET GOALS FOR TODAY

- ☐ CHECKED MY SUGAR EVERY 2 HOURS
- ☐ WAS MINDFUL WHEN EATING
- ☐ MEAL PREPPED
- ☐ CARB COUNTED FOOD

- ☐ VISUALIZED DAY OF GOOD BLOOD SUGARS
- ☐ TOOK 10 DEEP BREATHS
- ☐ PRE-BOLUSED MEALS
- ☐ SPENT TIME WITH LOVED ONES

- ☐ TOOK A WALK OUTSIDE
- ☐ _____
- ☐ _____
- ☐ _____

EXERCISE: _____

WATER: ⬜ ⬜ ⬜ ⬜ ⬜ ⬜ ⬜ ⬜ ⬜  TOTAL DAILY INSULIN: _____ UNITS

## THE NIGHT CAP

A PATTERN I RECOGNIZED WAS...

_____

_____

TOMORROW I WANT TO FOCUS MORE ON...

_____

_____

TODAY I CELEBRATE MYSELF BECAUSE...

_____

_____

# MORNING WORK IN | DATE: _____  S / M / T / W / T / F / S

## MINDSET PREP  I AM... _____

ONE THING I'M GRATEFUL FOR IS...

_____

ONE THING I DIDN'T DO YESTERDAY, BUT I WILL DO TODAY...

_____

## DAILY LOG

| TIME | BLOOD SUGAR | OUT OF RANGE (x) | INSULIN | C / F / P | NOTES / FOOD |
|------|-------------|------------------|---------|-----------|--------------|
|      |             |                  |         |           |              |
|      |             |                  |         |           |              |
|      |             |                  |         |           |              |
|      |             |                  |         |           |              |
|      |             |                  |         |           |              |
|      |             |                  |         |           |              |
|      |             |                  |         |           |              |
|      |             |                  |         |           |              |
|      |             |                  |         |           |              |
|      |             |                  |         |           |              |

# EVENING REFLECTION

"The most powerful relationship you will ever have is the relationship with yourself." – Steve Maraboli

| HOW I FELT | 1 (DISSATISFIED) | 2 | 3 (SO-SO) | 4 | 5 (ON FIRE!) |
|---|---|---|---|---|---|
| MOOD | | | | | |
| ENERGY | | | | | |
| BLOOD SUGAR | | | | | |
| NUTRITION | | | | | |
| MINDSET | | | | | |

## TODAY I...

☐ EXERCISED

☐ MEDITATED

☐ EXPRESSED GRATITUDE

☐ SET GOALS FOR TODAY

☐ CHECKED MY SUGAR EVERY 2 HOURS

☐ WAS MINDFUL WHEN EATING

☐ MEAL PREPPED

☐ CARB COUNTED FOOD

☐ VISUALIZED DAY OF GOOD BLOOD SUGARS

☐ TOOK 10 DEEP BREATHS

☐ PRE-BOLUSED MEALS

☐ SPENT TIME WITH LOVED ONES

☐ TOOK A WALK OUTSIDE

☐ _____

☐ _____

☐ _____

EXERCISE: _____

WATER: ☐ ☐ ☐ ☐ ☐ ☐ ☐ ☐ ☐ ☐      TOTAL DAILY INSULIN: _____ UNITS

## THE NIGHT CAP

A PATTERN I RECOGNIZED WAS...

_____

_____

TOMORROW I WANT TO FOCUS MORE ON...

_____

_____

TODAY I CELEBRATE MYSELF BECAUSE...

_____

_____

# MORNING WORK IN | DATE: _____ S / M / T / W / T / F / S

## MINDSET PREP

I AM... _____

ONE THING I'M GRATEFUL FOR IS...

_____

ONE THING I DIDN'T DO YESTERDAY, BUT I WILL DO TODAY...

_____

## DAILY LOG

| TIME | BLOOD SUGAR | OUT OF RANGE (x) | INSULIN | C / F / P | NOTES / FOOD |
|------|-------------|------------------|---------|-----------|--------------|
|      |             |                  |         |           |              |
|      |             |                  |         |           |              |
|      |             |                  |         |           |              |
|      |             |                  |         |           |              |
|      |             |                  |         |           |              |
|      |             |                  |         |           |              |
|      |             |                  |         |           |              |
|      |             |                  |         |           |              |
|      |             |                  |         |           |              |
|      |             |                  |         |           |              |

# EVENING REFLECTION | "When God throws a curveball, don't duck. You might miss something." – Movie *Extreme Days*

| HOW I FELT | 1 (DISSATISFIED) | 2 | 3 (SO-SO) | 4 | 5 (ON FIRE!) |
|---|---|---|---|---|---|
| MOOD | | | | | |
| ENERGY | | | | | |
| BLOOD SUGAR | | | | | |
| NUTRITION | | | | | |
| MINDSET | | | | | |

## TODAY I...

- ☐ EXERCISED
- ☐ CHECKED MY SUGAR EVERY 2 HOURS
- ☐ VISUALIZED DAY OF GOOD BLOOD SUGARS
- ☐ TOOK A WALK OUTSIDE

- ☐ MEDITATED
- ☐ WAS MINDFUL WHEN EATING
- ☐ TOOK 10 DEEP BREATHS
- ☐ _____

- ☐ EXPRESSED GRATITUDE
- ☐ MEAL PREPPED
- ☐ PRE-BOLUSED MEALS
- ☐ _____

- ☐ SET GOALS FOR TODAY
- ☐ CARB COUNTED FOOD
- ☐ SPENT TIME WITH LOVED ONES
- ☐ _____

EXERCISE: _____

WATER: ☐ ☐ ☐ ☐ ☐ ☐ ☐ ☐ ☐ ☐      TOTAL DAILY INSULIN: _____ UNITS

## THE NIGHT CAP

A PATTERN I RECOGNIZED WAS...

_____

_____

TOMORROW I WANT TO FOCUS MORE ON...

_____

_____

TODAY I CELEBRATE MYSELF BECAUSE...

_____

_____

# MORNING WORK IN | DATE: _____ S / M / T / W / T / F / S

## MINDSET PREP

I AM... _____

ONE THING I'M GRATEFUL FOR IS...

_____

ONE THING I DIDN'T DO YESTERDAY, BUT I WILL DO TODAY...

_____

## DAILY LOG

| TIME | BLOOD SUGAR | OUT OF RANGE (x) | INSULIN | C / F / P | NOTES / FOOD |
|------|-------------|------------------|---------|-----------|--------------|
|      |             |                  |         |           |              |
|      |             |                  |         |           |              |
|      |             |                  |         |           |              |
|      |             |                  |         |           |              |
|      |             |                  |         |           |              |
|      |             |                  |         |           |              |
|      |             |                  |         |           |              |
|      |             |                  |         |           |              |
|      |             |                  |         |           |              |

# EVENING REFLECTION

"Mindfulness isn't difficult, we just need to remember to do it."
– Sharon Salzberg

| HOW I FELT | 1 (DISSATISFIED) | 2 | 3 (SO-SO) | 4 | 5 (ON FIRE!) |
|---|---|---|---|---|---|
| MOOD | | | | | |
| ENERGY | | | | | |
| BLOOD SUGAR | | | | | |
| NUTRITION | | | | | |
| MINDSET | | | | | |

## TODAY I...

- ☐ EXERCISED
- ☐ MEDITATED
- ☐ EXPRESSED GRATITUDE
- ☐ SET GOALS FOR TODAY

- ☐ CHECKED MY SUGAR EVERY 2 HOURS
- ☐ WAS MINDFUL WHEN EATING
- ☐ MEAL PREPPED
- ☐ CARB COUNTED FOOD

- ☐ VISUALIZED DAY OF GOOD BLOOD SUGARS
- ☐ TOOK 10 DEEP BREATHS
- ☐ PRE-BOLUSED MEALS
- ☐ SPENT TIME WITH LOVED ONES

- ☐ TOOK A WALK OUTSIDE
- ☐ _____
- ☐ _____
- ☐ _____

EXERCISE: _____

WATER: ▽ ▽ ▽ ▽ ▽ ▽ ▽ ▽ ▽ ▽          TOTAL DAILY INSULIN: _____ UNITS

## THE NIGHT CAP

A PATTERN I RECOGNIZED WAS...

_____
_____

TOMORROW I WANT TO FOCUS MORE ON...

_____
_____

TODAY I CELEBRATE MYSELF BECAUSE...

_____
_____

# MORNING WORK IN | DATE: _____  S / M / T / W / T / F / S

I AM... _____

ONE THING I'M GRATEFUL FOR IS...

_____

ONE THING I DIDN'T DO YESTERDAY, BUT I WILL DO TODAY...

_____

## DAILY LOG

| TIME | BLOOD SUGAR | OUT OF RANGE (x) | INSULIN | C / F / P | NOTES / FOOD |
|------|-------------|------------------|---------|-----------|--------------|
|      |             |                  |         |           |              |
|      |             |                  |         |           |              |
|      |             |                  |         |           |              |
|      |             |                  |         |           |              |
|      |             |                  |         |           |              |
|      |             |                  |         |           |              |
|      |             |                  |         |           |              |
|      |             |                  |         |           |              |
|      |             |                  |         |           |              |
|      |             |                  |         |           |              |

# EVENING REFLECTION | *Lean into what makes you different.*

| HOW I FELT | 1<br>(DISSATISFIED) | 2 | 3<br>(SO-SO) | 4 | 5<br>(ON FIRE!) |
|---|---|---|---|---|---|
| MOOD | | | | | |
| ENERGY | | | | | |
| BLOOD SUGAR | | | | | |
| NUTRITION | | | | | |
| MINDSET | | | | | |

## TODAY I...

- ☐ EXERCISED
- ☐ MEDITATED
- ☐ EXPRESSED GRATITUDE
- ☐ SET GOALS FOR TODAY

- ☐ CHECKED MY SUGAR EVERY 2 HOURS
- ☐ WAS MINDFUL WHEN EATING
- ☐ MEAL PREPPED
- ☐ CARB COUNTED FOOD

- ☐ VISUALIZED DAY OF GOOD BLOOD SUGARS
- ☐ TOOK 10 DEEP BREATHS
- ☐ PRE-BOLUSED MEALS
- ☐ SPENT TIME WITH LOVED ONES

- ☐ TOOK A WALK OUTSIDE
- ☐ _____
- ☐ _____
- ☐ _____

EXERCISE: _____

WATER: 🥤 🥤 🥤 🥤 🥤 🥤 🥤 🥤 🥤 🥤     TOTAL DAILY INSULIN: _____ UNITS

## THE NIGHT CAP

A PATTERN I RECOGNIZED WAS...

_____

_____

TOMORROW I WANT TO FOCUS MORE ON...

_____

_____

TODAY I CELEBRATE MYSELF BECAUSE...

_____

_____

# MORNING WORK IN | DATE: _____  S / M / T / W / T / F / S

## MINDSET PREP

I AM... _____

ONE THING I'M GRATEFUL FOR IS...

_____

ONE THING I DIDN'T DO YESTERDAY, BUT I WILL DO TODAY...

_____

## DAILY LOG

| TIME | BLOOD SUGAR | OUT OF RANGE (x) | INSULIN | C / F / P | NOTES / FOOD |
|------|-------------|------------------|---------|-----------|--------------|
|      |             |                  |         |           |              |
|      |             |                  |         |           |              |
|      |             |                  |         |           |              |
|      |             |                  |         |           |              |
|      |             |                  |         |           |              |
|      |             |                  |         |           |              |
|      |             |                  |         |           |              |
|      |             |                  |         |           |              |
|      |             |                  |         |           |              |
|      |             |                  |         |           |              |

# EVENING REFLECTION

"Go all the way with it. Do not back off. Go all the damn way with what matters." – Ernest Hemingway

| HOW I FELT | 1 (DISSATISFIED) | 2 | 3 (SO-SO) | 4 | 5 (ON FIRE!) |
|---|---|---|---|---|---|
| MOOD | | | | | |
| ENERGY | | | | | |
| BLOOD SUGAR | | | | | |
| NUTRITION | | | | | |
| MINDSET | | | | | |

## TODAY I...

☐ EXERCISED    ☐ CHECKED MY SUGAR EVERY 2 HOURS    ☐ VISUALIZED DAY OF GOOD BLOOD SUGARS    ☐ TOOK A WALK OUTSIDE

☐ MEDITATED    ☐ WAS MINDFUL WHEN EATING    ☐ TOOK 10 DEEP BREATHS    ☐ _____

☐ EXPRESSED GRATITUDE    ☐ MEAL PREPPED    ☐ PRE-BOLUSED MEALS    ☐ _____

☐ SET GOALS FOR TODAY    ☐ CARB COUNTED FOOD    ☐ SPENT TIME WITH LOVED ONES    ☐ _____

EXERCISE: _____

WATER: ☐ ☐ ☐ ☐ ☐ ☐ ☐ ☐ ☐ ☐    TOTAL DAILY INSULIN: _____ UNITS

## THE NIGHT CAP

A PATTERN I RECOGNIZED WAS...

_____

_____

TOMORROW I WANT TO FOCUS MORE ON...

_____

_____

TODAY I CELEBRATE MYSELF BECAUSE...

_____

_____

# MORNING WORK IN | DATE: _____ S / M / T / W / T / F / S

## MINDSET PREP

I AM... _____

ONE THING I'M GRATEFUL FOR IS...

_____

ONE THING I DIDN'T DO YESTERDAY, BUT I WILL DO TODAY...

_____

## DAILY LOG

| TIME | BLOOD SUGAR | OUT OF RANGE (x) | INSULIN | C / F / P | NOTES / FOOD |
|------|------|------|------|------|------|
|  |  |  |  |  |  |
|  |  |  |  |  |  |
|  |  |  |  |  |  |
|  |  |  |  |  |  |
|  |  |  |  |  |  |
|  |  |  |  |  |  |
|  |  |  |  |  |  |
|  |  |  |  |  |  |
|  |  |  |  |  |  |

# EVENING REFLECTION

**JOURNAL PROMPT:**
If you had to write a letter of gratitude to your diabetes,
what would it say?

| HOW I FELT | 1 (DISSATISFIED) | 2 | 3 (SO-SO) | 4 | 5 (ON FIRE!) |
|---|---|---|---|---|---|
| MOOD | | | | | |
| ENERGY | | | | | |
| BLOOD SUGAR | | | | | |
| NUTRITION | | | | | |
| MINDSET | | | | | |

## TODAY I...

- ☐ EXERCISED
- ☐ MEDITATED
- ☐ EXPRESSED GRATITUDE
- ☐ SET GOALS FOR TODAY

- ☐ CHECKED MY SUGAR EVERY 2 HOURS
- ☐ WAS MINDFUL WHEN EATING
- ☐ MEAL PREPPED
- ☐ CARB COUNTED FOOD

- ☐ VISUALIZED DAY OF GOOD BLOOD SUGARS
- ☐ TOOK 10 DEEP BREATHS
- ☐ PRE-BOLUSED MEALS
- ☐ SPENT TIME WITH LOVED ONES

- ☐ TOOK A WALK OUTSIDE
- ☐ _____
- ☐ _____
- ☐ _____

EXERCISE: _____

WATER: ☐ ☐ ☐ ☐ ☐ ☐ ☐ ☐ ☐ ☐     TOTAL DAILY INSULIN: _____ UNITS

## THE NIGHT CAP

A PATTERN I RECOGNIZED WAS...

_____

_____

TOMORROW I WANT TO FOCUS MORE ON...

_____

_____

TODAY I CELEBRATE MYSELF BECAUSE...

_____

_____

# MORNING WORK IN | DATE: _____

## MINDSET PREP    I AM... _____

ONE THING I'M GRATEFUL FOR IS...

_____

ONE THING I DIDN'T DO YESTERDAY, BUT I WILL DO TODAY...

_____

## DAILY LOG

| TIME | BLOOD SUGAR | OUT OF RANGE (x) | INSULIN | C / F / P | NOTES / FOOD |
|------|-------------|------------------|---------|-----------|--------------|
|      |             |                  |         |           |              |
|      |             |                  |         |           |              |
|      |             |                  |         |           |              |
|      |             |                  |         |           |              |
|      |             |                  |         |           |              |
|      |             |                  |         |           |              |
|      |             |                  |         |           |              |
|      |             |                  |         |           |              |
|      |             |                  |         |           |              |

# EVENING REFLECTION

"I love listening. It's one of the only spaces where you can be still and be moved, both at the same time." – Nayyirah Waheed

## HOW I FELT

|  | 1 (DISSATISFIED) | 2 | 3 (SO-SO) | 4 | 5 (ON FIRE!) |
|---|---|---|---|---|---|
| MOOD | | | | | |
| ENERGY | | | | | |
| BLOOD SUGAR | | | | | |
| NUTRITION | | | | | |
| MINDSET | | | | | |

## TODAY I...

- [ ] EXERCISED
- [ ] MEDITATED
- [ ] EXPRESSED GRATITUDE
- [ ] SET GOALS FOR TODAY

- [ ] CHECKED MY SUGAR EVERY 2 HOURS
- [ ] WAS MINDFUL WHEN EATING
- [ ] MEAL PREPPED
- [ ] CARB COUNTED FOOD

- [ ] VISUALIZED DAY OF GOOD BLOOD SUGARS
- [ ] TOOK 10 DEEP BREATHS
- [ ] PRE-BOLUSED MEALS
- [ ] SPENT TIME WITH LOVED ONES

- [ ] TOOK A WALK OUTSIDE
- [ ] _____
- [ ] _____
- [ ] _____

EXERCISE: _____

WATER: ⊔ ⊔ ⊔ ⊔ ⊔ ⊔ ⊔ ⊔ ⊔ ⊔          TOTAL DAILY INSULIN: _____ UNITS

## THE NIGHT CAP

A PATTERN I RECOGNIZED WAS...

_____
_____

TOMORROW I WANT TO FOCUS MORE ON...

_____
_____

TODAY I CELEBRATE MYSELF BECAUSE...

_____
_____

# MORNING WORK IN | DATE: _____  S / M / T / W / T / F / S

## MINDSET PREP          I AM... _____

ONE THING I'M GRATEFUL FOR IS...

_____

ONE THING I DIDN'T DO YESTERDAY, BUT I WILL DO TODAY...

_____

## DAILY LOG

| TIME | BLOOD SUGAR | OUT OF RANGE (x) | INSULIN | C / F / P | NOTES / FOOD |
|---|---|---|---|---|---|
|  |  |  |  |  |  |
|  |  |  |  |  |  |
|  |  |  |  |  |  |
|  |  |  |  |  |  |
|  |  |  |  |  |  |
|  |  |  |  |  |  |
|  |  |  |  |  |  |
|  |  |  |  |  |  |
|  |  |  |  |  |  |

# EVENING REFLECTION

"It is not the mountain we conquer but ourselves."
– Edmund Hillary

| HOW I FELT | 1 (DISSATISFIED) | 2 | 3 (SO-SO) | 4 | 5 (ON FIRE!) |
|---|---|---|---|---|---|
| MOOD | | | | | |
| ENERGY | | | | | |
| BLOOD SUGAR | | | | | |
| NUTRITION | | | | | |
| MINDSET | | | | | |

## TODAY I...

- ☐ EXERCISED
- ☐ MEDITATED
- ☐ EXPRESSED GRATITUDE
- ☐ SET GOALS FOR TODAY

- ☐ CHECKED MY SUGAR EVERY 2 HOURS
- ☐ WAS MINDFUL WHEN EATING
- ☐ MEAL PREPPED
- ☐ CARB COUNTED FOOD

- ☐ VISUALIZED DAY OF GOOD BLOOD SUGARS
- ☐ TOOK 10 DEEP BREATHS
- ☐ PRE-BOLUSED MEALS
- ☐ SPENT TIME WITH LOVED ONES

- ☐ TOOK A WALK OUTSIDE
- ☐ _____
- ☐ _____
- ☐ _____

EXERCISE: _____

WATER: ⛌ ⛌ ⛌ ⛌ ⛌ ⛌ ⛌ ⛌ ⛌ ⛌      TOTAL DAILY INSULIN: _____ UNITS

## THE NIGHT CAP

A PATTERN I RECOGNIZED WAS...

_____

_____

TOMORROW I WANT TO FOCUS MORE ON...

_____

_____

TODAY I CELEBRATE MYSELF BECAUSE...

_____

_____

# MORNING WORK IN | DATE: _____ S / M / T / W / T / F / S

## MINDSET PREP

I AM... _____

ONE THING I'M GRATEFUL FOR IS...

_____

ONE THING I DIDN'T DO YESTERDAY, BUT I WILL DO TODAY...

_____

## DAILY LOG

| TIME | BLOOD SUGAR | OUT OF RANGE (x) | INSULIN | C / F / P | NOTES / FOOD |
|------|-------------|------------------|---------|-----------|--------------|
|      |             |                  |         |           |              |
|      |             |                  |         |           |              |
|      |             |                  |         |           |              |
|      |             |                  |         |           |              |
|      |             |                  |         |           |              |
|      |             |                  |         |           |              |
|      |             |                  |         |           |              |
|      |             |                  |         |           |              |
|      |             |                  |         |           |              |

# EVENING REFLECTION | "It is always our responsibility to surround ourselves with what we need most." – LNB

| HOW I FELT | 1 (DISSATISFIED) | 2 | 3 (SO-SO) | 4 | 5 (ON FIRE!) |
|---|---|---|---|---|---|
| MOOD | | | | | |
| ENERGY | | | | | |
| BLOOD SUGAR | | | | | |
| NUTRITION | | | | | |
| MINDSET | | | | | |

## TODAY I...

- ☐ EXERCISED
- ☐ MEDITATED
- ☐ EXPRESSED GRATITUDE
- ☐ SET GOALS FOR TODAY

- ☐ CHECKED MY SUGAR EVERY 2 HOURS
- ☐ WAS MINDFUL WHEN EATING
- ☐ MEAL PREPPED
- ☐ CARB COUNTED FOOD

- ☐ VISUALIZED DAY OF GOOD BLOOD SUGARS
- ☐ TOOK 10 DEEP BREATHS
- ☐ PRE-BOLUSED MEALS
- ☐ SPENT TIME WITH LOVED ONES

- ☐ TOOK A WALK OUTSIDE
- ☐ _____
- ☐ _____
- ☐ _____

EXERCISE: _____

WATER: ⬜ ⬜ ⬜ ⬜ ⬜ ⬜ ⬜ ⬜ ⬜ ⬜    TOTAL DAILY INSULIN: _____ UNITS

## THE NIGHT CAP

A PATTERN I RECOGNIZED WAS...

_____

_____

TOMORROW I WANT TO FOCUS MORE ON...

_____

_____

TODAY I CELEBRATE MYSELF BECAUSE...

_____

_____

# MORNING WORK IN

DATE: _____  S / M / T / W / T / F / S

## MINDSET PREP

I AM... _____

ONE THING I'M GRATEFUL FOR IS...

_____

ONE THING I DIDN'T DO YESTERDAY, BUT I WILL DO TODAY...

_____

## DAILY LOG

| TIME | BLOOD SUGAR | OUT OF RANGE (x) | INSULIN | C / F / P | NOTES / FOOD |
|------|-------------|------------------|---------|-----------|--------------|
|      |             |                  |         |           |              |
|      |             |                  |         |           |              |
|      |             |                  |         |           |              |
|      |             |                  |         |           |              |
|      |             |                  |         |           |              |
|      |             |                  |         |           |              |
|      |             |                  |         |           |              |
|      |             |                  |         |           |              |
|      |             |                  |         |           |              |

# EVENING REFLECTION

"Nothing can dim the light that shines from within."
– Maya Angelou

| HOW I FELT | 1 (DISSATISFIED) | 2 | 3 (SO-SO) | 4 | 5 (ON FIRE!) |
|---|---|---|---|---|---|
| MOOD | | | | | |
| ENERGY | | | | | |
| BLOOD SUGAR | | | | | |
| NUTRITION | | | | | |
| MINDSET | | | | | |

## TODAY I...

☐ EXERCISED
☐ MEDITATED
☐ EXPRESSED GRATITUDE
☐ SET GOALS FOR TODAY

☐ CHECKED MY SUGAR EVERY 2 HOURS
☐ WAS MINDFUL WHEN EATING
☐ MEAL PREPPED
☐ CARB COUNTED FOOD

☐ VISUALIZED DAY OF GOOD BLOOD SUGARS
☐ TOOK 10 DEEP BREATHS
☐ PRE-BOLUSED MEALS
☐ SPENT TIME WITH LOVED ONES

☐ TOOK A WALK OUTSIDE
☐ _____
☐ _____
☐ _____

EXERCISE: _____

WATER: ☐ ☐ ☐ ☐ ☐ ☐ ☐ ☐ ☐ ☐    TOTAL DAILY INSULIN: _____ UNITS

## THE NIGHT CAP

A PATTERN I RECOGNIZED WAS...

_____

_____

TOMORROW I WANT TO FOCUS MORE ON...

_____

_____

TODAY I CELEBRATE MYSELF BECAUSE...

_____

_____

# MORNING WORK IN | DATE: _____ S / M / T / W / T / F / S

## MINDSET PREP

I AM... _____

ONE THING I'M GRATEFUL FOR IS...

_____

ONE THING I DIDN'T DO YESTERDAY, BUT I WILL DO TODAY...

_____

## DAILY LOG

| TIME | BLOOD SUGAR | OUT OF RANGE (x) | INSULIN | C / F / P | NOTES / FOOD |
|------|-------------|------------------|---------|-----------|--------------|
|      |             |                  |         |           |              |
|      |             |                  |         |           |              |
|      |             |                  |         |           |              |
|      |             |                  |         |           |              |
|      |             |                  |         |           |              |
|      |             |                  |         |           |              |
|      |             |                  |         |           |              |
|      |             |                  |         |           |              |
|      |             |                  |         |           |              |

# EVENING REFLECTION | "Where attention goes energy flows." – James Redfield

| HOW I FELT | 1 (DISSATISFIED) | 2 | 3 (SO-SO) | 4 | 5 (ON FIRE!) |
|---|---|---|---|---|---|
| MOOD | | | | | |
| ENERGY | | | | | |
| BLOOD SUGAR | | | | | |
| NUTRITION | | | | | |
| MINDSET | | | | | |

## TODAY I...

☐ EXERCISED

☐ MEDITATED

☐ EXPRESSED GRATITUDE

☐ SET GOALS FOR TODAY

☐ CHECKED MY SUGAR EVERY 2 HOURS

☐ WAS MINDFUL WHEN EATING

☐ MEAL PREPPED

☐ CARB COUNTED FOOD

☐ VISUALIZED DAY OF GOOD BLOOD SUGARS

☐ TOOK 10 DEEP BREATHS

☐ PRE-BOLUSED MEALS

☐ SPENT TIME WITH LOVED ONES

☐ TOOK A WALK OUTSIDE

☐ _____

☐ _____

☐ _____

EXERCISE: _____

WATER: ⬜ ⬜ ⬜ ⬜ ⬜ ⬜ ⬜ ⬜ ⬜ ⬜    TOTAL DAILY INSULIN: _____ UNITS

## THE NIGHT CAP

A PATTERN I RECOGNIZED WAS...

_____

_____

TOMORROW I WANT TO FOCUS MORE ON...

_____

_____

TODAY I CELEBRATE MYSELF BECAUSE...

_____

_____

# MONTH 01 REVIEW + REFLECT

## DIABETES MANAGEMENT SPECIFICS

1. My updated average fasting blood sugar (waking up)? _____

2. My updated current basal insulin:

| TIME OF DAY | MY BASAL |
|---|---|
| 12:00am | |
| | |
| | |
| | |
| | |
| | |
| | |

3. My updated current Insulin: Carb Ratio/s:

| TIME OF DAY | MY ICR |
|---|---|
| 12:00am | |
| | |
| | |
| | |
| | |
| | |
| | |

4. My updated current Insulin Sensitivity Factor/s:

| TIME OF DAY | MY ISF |
|---|---|
| 12:00am | |
| | |
| | |
| | |
| | |
| | |
| | |

5. What actions over the last month have you recognized **best** serve your blood sugars?

_____

_____

6. What actions over the last month have you recognized **least** serve your blood sugars?

_____

_____

# MIND / BODY / SOUL

1. What changes in your mind, body, or soul are you most proud of so far?

_____

_____

_____

_____

_____

2. What challenges came up for you this month? Were they in or out of your control? What can you learn from them?

_____

_____

_____

_____

_____

# REFINING MY GOALS

Reflect on the three overarching goals you set at the start of the journal. Rewrite (or update if necessary) your 3 month goals below with new action steps beneath each.

Goal #1: _____

1 SMART Action Step: _____

Goal #2: _____

1 SMART Action Step: _____

Goal #3: _____

1 SMART Action Step: _____

# THE MIND HAS TO ARRIVE AT THE DESTINATION BEFORE THE BODY DOES

# MONTH 02

## WEEKLY CHALLENGE

WEEK 01 _____

_____ ☐ DONE

WEEK 02 _____

_____ ☐ DONE

WEEK 03 _____

_____ ☐ DONE

WEEK 04 _____

_____ ☐ DONE

# MORNING WORK IN | DATE: _____  S / M / T / W / T / F / S

## MINDSET PREP

I AM... _____

ONE THING I'M GRATEFUL FOR IS...

_____

ONE THING I DIDN'T DO YESTERDAY, BUT I WILL DO TODAY...

_____

## DAILY LOG

| TIME | BLOOD SUGAR | OUT OF RANGE (X) | INSULIN | C / F / P | NOTES / FOOD |
|------|-------------|------------------|---------|-----------|--------------|
|      |             |                  |         |           |              |
|      |             |                  |         |           |              |
|      |             |                  |         |           |              |
|      |             |                  |         |           |              |
|      |             |                  |         |           |              |
|      |             |                  |         |           |              |
|      |             |                  |         |           |              |
|      |             |                  |         |           |              |
|      |             |                  |         |           |              |

# EVENING REFLECTION | "If you learn from defeat, you haven't really lost." – Zig Ziglar

| HOW I FELT | 1 (DISSATISFIED) | 2 | 3 (SO-SO) | 4 | 5 (ON FIRE!) |
|---|---|---|---|---|---|
| MOOD | | | | | |
| ENERGY | | | | | |
| BLOOD SUGAR | | | | | |
| NUTRITION | | | | | |
| MINDSET | | | | | |

## TODAY I...

☐ EXERCISED  ☐ CHECKED MY SUGAR EVERY 2 HOURS  ☐ VISUALIZED DAY OF GOOD BLOOD SUGARS  ☐ TOOK A WALK OUTSIDE

☐ MEDITATED  ☐ WAS MINDFUL WHEN EATING  ☐ TOOK 10 DEEP BREATHS  ☐ _____

☐ EXPRESSED GRATITUDE  ☐ MEAL PREPPED  ☐ PRE-BOLUSED MEALS  ☐ _____

☐ SET GOALS FOR TODAY  ☐ CARB COUNTED FOOD  ☐ SPENT TIME WITH LOVED ONES  ☐ _____

EXERCISE: _____

WATER: ▭ ▭ ▭ ▭ ▭ ▭ ▭ ▭ ▭ ▭    TOTAL DAILY INSULIN: _____ UNITS

## THE NIGHT CAP

A PATTERN I RECOGNIZED WAS...

_____

_____

TOMORROW I WANT TO FOCUS MORE ON...

_____

_____

TODAY I CELEBRATE MYSELF BECAUSE...

_____

_____

# MORNING WORK IN | DATE: _____ S / M / T / W / T / F / S

## MINDSET PREP

I AM... _____

ONE THING I'M GRATEFUL FOR IS...

_____

ONE THING I DIDN'T DO YESTERDAY, BUT I WILL DO TODAY...

_____

## DAILY LOG

| TIME | BLOOD SUGAR | OUT OF RANGE (x) | INSULIN | C / F / P | NOTES / FOOD |
|------|-------------|------------------|---------|-----------|--------------|
|      |             |                  |         |           |              |
|      |             |                  |         |           |              |
|      |             |                  |         |           |              |
|      |             |                  |         |           |              |
|      |             |                  |         |           |              |
|      |             |                  |         |           |              |
|      |             |                  |         |           |              |
|      |             |                  |         |           |              |
|      |             |                  |         |           |              |
|      |             |                  |         |           |              |

# EVENING REFLECTION | "The barrier isn't the body, it's the mind." - David Goggins

| HOW I FELT | 1 (DISSATISFIED) | 2 | 3 (SO-SO) | 4 | 5 (ON FIRE!) |
|---|---|---|---|---|---|
| MOOD | | | | | |
| ENERGY | | | | | |
| BLOOD SUGAR | | | | | |
| NUTRITION | | | | | |
| MINDSET | | | | | |

## TODAY I...

- ☐ EXERCISED
- ☐ CHECKED MY SUGAR EVERY 2 HOURS
- ☐ VISUALIZED DAY OF GOOD BLOOD SUGARS
- ☐ TOOK A WALK OUTSIDE

- ☐ MEDITATED
- ☐ WAS MINDFUL WHEN EATING
- ☐ TOOK 10 DEEP BREATHS
- ☐ _____

- ☐ EXPRESSED GRATITUDE
- ☐ MEAL PREPPED
- ☐ PRE-BOLUSED MEALS
- ☐ _____

- ☐ SET GOALS FOR TODAY
- ☐ CARB COUNTED FOOD
- ☐ SPENT TIME WITH LOVED ONES
- ☐ _____

EXERCISE: _____

WATER: ⊔ ⊔ ⊔ ⊔ ⊔ ⊔ ⊔ ⊔ ⊔ ⊔     TOTAL DAILY INSULIN: _____ UNITS

## THE NIGHT CAP

A PATTERN I RECOGNIZED WAS...

_____

_____

TOMORROW I WANT TO FOCUS MORE ON...

_____

_____

TODAY I CELEBRATE MYSELF BECAUSE...

_____

_____

# MORNING WORK IN | DATE: _____ \quad S / M / T / W / T / F / S

## MINDSET PREP

I AM... _____

ONE THING I'M GRATEFUL FOR IS...

_____

ONE THING I DIDN'T DO YESTERDAY, BUT I WILL DO TODAY...

_____

## DAILY LOG

| TIME | BLOOD SUGAR | OUT OF RANGE (x) | INSULIN | C / F / P | NOTES / FOOD |
|------|-------------|------------------|---------|-----------|--------------|
|      |             |                  |         |           |              |
|      |             |                  |         |           |              |
|      |             |                  |         |           |              |
|      |             |                  |         |           |              |
|      |             |                  |         |           |              |
|      |             |                  |         |           |              |
|      |             |                  |         |           |              |
|      |             |                  |         |           |              |
|      |             |                  |         |           |              |
|      |             |                  |         |           |              |

# EVENING REFLECTION

"Perspective shifts will unlock more than smartness will."
– Astro Teller

| HOW I FELT | 1 (DISSATISFIED) | 2 | 3 (SO-SO) | 4 | 5 (ON FIRE!) |
|---|---|---|---|---|---|
| MOOD | | | | | |
| ENERGY | | | | | |
| BLOOD SUGAR | | | | | |
| NUTRITION | | | | | |
| MINDSET | | | | | |

## TODAY I...

☐ EXERCISED

☐ MEDITATED

☐ EXPRESSED GRATITUDE

☐ SET GOALS FOR TODAY

☐ CHECKED MY SUGAR EVERY 2 HOURS

☐ WAS MINDFUL WHEN EATING

☐ MEAL PREPPED

☐ CARB COUNTED FOOD

☐ VISUALIZED DAY OF GOOD BLOOD SUGARS

☐ TOOK 10 DEEP BREATHS

☐ PRE-BOLUSED MEALS

☐ SPENT TIME WITH LOVED ONES

☐ TOOK A WALK OUTSIDE

☐ _____

☐ _____

☐ _____

EXERCISE: _____

WATER: ☐ ☐ ☐ ☐ ☐ ☐ ☐ ☐ ☐ ☐          TOTAL DAILY INSULIN: _____ UNITS

## THE NIGHT CAP

A PATTERN I RECOGNIZED WAS...

_____

_____

TOMORROW I WANT TO FOCUS MORE ON...

_____

_____

TODAY I CELEBRATE MYSELF BECAUSE...

_____

_____

# MORNING WORK IN

DATE: _____

## MINDSET PREP

I AM... _____

ONE THING I'M GRATEFUL FOR IS...

_____

ONE THING I DIDN'T DO YESTERDAY, BUT I WILL DO TODAY...

_____

## DAILY LOG

| TIME | BLOOD SUGAR | OUT OF RANGE (x) | INSULIN | C / F / P | NOTES / FOOD |
|------|-------------|------------------|---------|-----------|--------------|
|      |             |                  |         |           |              |
|      |             |                  |         |           |              |
|      |             |                  |         |           |              |
|      |             |                  |         |           |              |
|      |             |                  |         |           |              |
|      |             |                  |         |           |              |
|      |             |                  |         |           |              |
|      |             |                  |         |           |              |
|      |             |                  |         |           |              |

# EVENING REFLECTION

"Never be satisfied with less than your very best effort.
If you strive for the top and miss, you'll still beat the pack."
– Gerald R. Ford

| HOW I FELT | 1 (DISSATISFIED) | 2 | 3 (SO-SO) | 4 | 5 (ON FIRE!) |
|---|---|---|---|---|---|
| MOOD | | | | | |
| ENERGY | | | | | |
| BLOOD SUGAR | | | | | |
| NUTRITION | | | | | |
| MINDSET | | | | | |

## TODAY I...

☐ EXERCISED

☐ MEDITATED

☐ EXPRESSED GRATITUDE

☐ SET GOALS FOR TODAY

☐ CHECKED MY SUGAR EVERY 2 HOURS

☐ WAS MINDFUL WHEN EATING

☐ MEAL PREPPED

☐ CARB COUNTED FOOD

☐ VISUALIZED DAY OF GOOD BLOOD SUGARS

☐ TOOK 10 DEEP BREATHS

☐ PRE-BOLUSED MEALS

☐ SPENT TIME WITH LOVED ONES

☐ TOOK A WALK OUTSIDE

☐ _____

☐ _____

☐ _____

EXERCISE: _____

WATER: ☐ ☐ ☐ ☐ ☐ ☐ ☐ ☐ ☐ ☐     TOTAL DAILY INSULIN: _____ UNITS

## THE NIGHT CAP

A PATTERN I RECOGNIZED WAS...

_____

_____

TOMORROW I WANT TO FOCUS MORE ON...

_____

_____

TODAY I CELEBRATE MYSELF BECAUSE...

_____

_____

# MORNING WORK IN

DATE: _____  S / M / T / W / T / F / S

I AM... _____

ONE THING I'M GRATEFUL FOR IS...

_____

ONE THING I DIDN'T DO YESTERDAY, BUT I WILL DO TODAY...

_____

## DAILY LOG

| TIME | BLOOD SUGAR | OUT OF RANGE (x) | INSULIN | C / F / P | NOTES / FOOD |
|------|-------------|------------------|---------|-----------|--------------|
|      |             |                  |         |           |              |
|      |             |                  |         |           |              |
|      |             |                  |         |           |              |
|      |             |                  |         |           |              |
|      |             |                  |         |           |              |
|      |             |                  |         |           |              |
|      |             |                  |         |           |              |
|      |             |                  |         |           |              |
|      |             |                  |         |           |              |
|      |             |                  |         |           |              |

# EVENING REFLECTION

*An arrow can only be shot by pulling it backward. So when life is dragging you back with difficulties, it means that it's going to launch you into something great. So just focus, and keep aiming.*

## HOW I FELT

| | 1 (DISSATISFIED) | 2 | 3 (SO-SO) | 4 | 5 (ON FIRE!) |
|---|---|---|---|---|---|
| MOOD | | | | | |
| ENERGY | | | | | |
| BLOOD SUGAR | | | | | |
| NUTRITION | | | | | |
| MINDSET | | | | | |

## TODAY I...

☐ EXERCISED    ☐ CHECKED MY SUGAR EVERY 2 HOURS    ☐ VISUALIZED DAY OF GOOD BLOOD SUGARS    ☐ TOOK A WALK OUTSIDE

☐ MEDITATED    ☐ WAS MINDFUL WHEN EATING    ☐ TOOK 10 DEEP BREATHS    ☐ _____

☐ EXPRESSED GRATITUDE    ☐ MEAL PREPPED    ☐ PRE-BOLUSED MEALS    ☐ _____

☐ SET GOALS FOR TODAY    ☐ CARB COUNTED FOOD    ☐ SPENT TIME WITH LOVED ONES    ☐ _____

EXERCISE: _____

WATER: ▽ ▽ ▽ ▽ ▽ ▽ ▽ ▽ ▽ ▽        TOTAL DAILY INSULIN: _____ UNITS

## THE NIGHT CAP

A PATTERN I RECOGNIZED WAS...

_____

_____

TOMORROW I WANT TO FOCUS MORE ON...

_____

_____

TODAY I CELEBRATE MYSELF BECAUSE...

_____

_____

# MORNING WORK IN | DATE: _____ S / M / T / W / T / F / S

## MINDSET PREP

I AM... _____

ONE THING I'M GRATEFUL FOR IS...

_____

ONE THING I DIDN'T DO YESTERDAY, BUT I WILL DO TODAY...

_____

## DAILY LOG

| TIME | BLOOD SUGAR | OUT OF RANGE (x) | INSULIN | C / F / P | NOTES / FOOD |
|------|-------------|------------------|---------|-----------|--------------|
|      |             |                  |         |           |              |
|      |             |                  |         |           |              |
|      |             |                  |         |           |              |
|      |             |                  |         |           |              |
|      |             |                  |         |           |              |
|      |             |                  |         |           |              |
|      |             |                  |         |           |              |
|      |             |                  |         |           |              |
|      |             |                  |         |           |              |

# EVENING REFLECTION

**JOURNAL PROMPT:**
What is one thing you will work on today that you've been putting off?

## HOW I FELT

| | 1 (DISSATISFIED) | 2 | 3 (SO-SO) | 4 | 5 (ON FIRE!) |
|---|---|---|---|---|---|
| MOOD | | | | | |
| ENERGY | | | | | |
| BLOOD SUGAR | | | | | |
| NUTRITION | | | | | |
| MINDSET | | | | | |

## TODAY I...

- ☐ EXERCISED
- ☐ CHECKED MY SUGAR EVERY 2 HOURS
- ☐ VISUALIZED DAY OF GOOD BLOOD SUGARS
- ☐ TOOK A WALK OUTSIDE

- ☐ MEDITATED
- ☐ WAS MINDFUL WHEN EATING
- ☐ TOOK 10 DEEP BREATHS
- ☐ _____

- ☐ EXPRESSED GRATITUDE
- ☐ MEAL PREPPED
- ☐ PRE-BOLUSED MEALS
- ☐ _____

- ☐ SET GOALS FOR TODAY
- ☐ CARB COUNTED FOOD
- ☐ SPENT TIME WITH LOVED ONES
- ☐ _____

EXERCISE: _____

WATER: ☐ ☐ ☐ ☐ ☐ ☐ ☐ ☐ ☐ ☐     TOTAL DAILY INSULIN: _____ UNITS

## THE NIGHT CAP

A PATTERN I RECOGNIZED WAS...

_____
_____

TOMORROW I WANT TO FOCUS MORE ON...

_____
_____

TODAY I CELEBRATE MYSELF BECAUSE...

_____
_____

# MORNING WORK IN | DATE: _____ S / M / T / W / T / F / S

## MINDSET PREP

I AM... _____

ONE THING I'M GRATEFUL FOR IS...

_____

ONE THING I DIDN'T DO YESTERDAY, BUT I WILL DO TODAY...

_____

## DAILY LOG

| TIME | BLOOD SUGAR | OUT OF RANGE (x) | INSULIN | C / F / P | NOTES / FOOD |
|------|-------------|------------------|---------|-----------|--------------|
|      |             |                  |         |           |              |
|      |             |                  |         |           |              |
|      |             |                  |         |           |              |
|      |             |                  |         |           |              |
|      |             |                  |         |           |              |
|      |             |                  |         |           |              |
|      |             |                  |         |           |              |
|      |             |                  |         |           |              |
|      |             |                  |         |           |              |

# EVENING REFLECTION | "We are what we repeatedly do. Therefore, excellence is not an act, but a habit." – Aristotle

## HOW I FELT

| | 1 (DISSATISFIED) | 2 | 3 (SO-SO) | 4 | 5 (ON FIRE!) |
|---|---|---|---|---|---|
| MOOD | | | | | |
| ENERGY | | | | | |
| BLOOD SUGAR | | | | | |
| NUTRITION | | | | | |
| MINDSET | | | | | |

## TODAY I...

- [ ] EXERCISED
- [ ] MEDITATED
- [ ] EXPRESSED GRATITUDE
- [ ] SET GOALS FOR TODAY

- [ ] CHECKED MY SUGAR EVERY 2 HOURS
- [ ] WAS MINDFUL WHEN EATING
- [ ] MEAL PREPPED
- [ ] CARB COUNTED FOOD

- [ ] VISUALIZED DAY OF GOOD BLOOD SUGARS
- [ ] TOOK 10 DEEP BREATHS
- [ ] PRE-BOLUSED MEALS
- [ ] SPENT TIME WITH LOVED ONES

- [ ] TOOK A WALK OUTSIDE
- [ ] _____
- [ ] _____
- [ ] _____

EXERCISE: _____

WATER: 🥤🥤🥤🥤🥤🥤🥤🥤🥤🥤          TOTAL DAILY INSULIN: _____ UNITS

## THE NIGHT CAP

A PATTERN I RECOGNIZED WAS...

_____

_____

TOMORROW I WANT TO FOCUS MORE ON...

_____

_____

TODAY I CELEBRATE MYSELF BECAUSE...

_____

_____

# MORNING WORK IN | DATE: _____  S / M / T / W / T / F / S

## MINDSET PREP

I AM... _____

ONE THING I'M GRATEFUL FOR IS...

_____

ONE THING I DIDN'T DO YESTERDAY, BUT I WILL DO TODAY...

_____

## DAILY LOG

| TIME | BLOOD SUGAR | OUT OF RANGE (x) | INSULIN | C / F / P | NOTES / FOOD |
|------|-------------|------------------|---------|-----------|--------------|
|      |             |                  |         |           |              |
|      |             |                  |         |           |              |
|      |             |                  |         |           |              |
|      |             |                  |         |           |              |
|      |             |                  |         |           |              |
|      |             |                  |         |           |              |
|      |             |                  |         |           |              |
|      |             |                  |         |           |              |
|      |             |                  |         |           |              |

# EVENING REFLECTION | "You are the sky. Everything else is just the weather."
– Pema Chödrön

| HOW I FELT | 1 (DISSATISFIED) | 2 | 3 (SO-SO) | 4 | 5 (ON FIRE!) |
|---|---|---|---|---|---|
| MOOD | | | | | |
| ENERGY | | | | | |
| BLOOD SUGAR | | | | | |
| NUTRITION | | | | | |
| MINDSET | | | | | |

## TODAY I...

- [ ] EXERCISED
- [ ] MEDITATED
- [ ] EXPRESSED GRATITUDE
- [ ] SET GOALS FOR TODAY

- [ ] CHECKED MY SUGAR EVERY 2 HOURS
- [ ] WAS MINDFUL WHEN EATING
- [ ] MEAL PREPPED
- [ ] CARB COUNTED FOOD

- [ ] VISUALIZED DAY OF GOOD BLOOD SUGARS
- [ ] TOOK 10 DEEP BREATHS
- [ ] PRE-BOLUSED MEALS
- [ ] SPENT TIME WITH LOVED ONES

- [ ] TOOK A WALK OUTSIDE
- [ ] _____
- [ ] _____
- [ ] _____

EXERCISE: _____

WATER: 🥤🥤🥤🥤🥤🥤🥤🥤🥤🥤     TOTAL DAILY INSULIN: _____ UNITS

## THE NIGHT CAP

A PATTERN I RECOGNIZED WAS...

_____

_____

TOMORROW I WANT TO FOCUS MORE ON...

_____

_____

TODAY I CELEBRATE MYSELF BECAUSE...

_____

_____

# MORNING WORK IN

## MINDSET PREP

I AM... _____

ONE THING I'M GRATEFUL FOR IS...

_____

ONE THING I DIDN'T DO YESTERDAY, BUT I WILL DO TODAY...

_____

## DAILY LOG

| TIME | BLOOD SUGAR | OUT OF RANGE (x) | INSULIN | C / F / P | NOTES / FOOD |
|------|-------------|------------------|---------|-----------|--------------|
|      |             |                  |         |           |              |
|      |             |                  |         |           |              |
|      |             |                  |         |           |              |
|      |             |                  |         |           |              |
|      |             |                  |         |           |              |
|      |             |                  |         |           |              |
|      |             |                  |         |           |              |
|      |             |                  |         |           |              |
|      |             |                  |         |           |              |

# EVENING REFLECTION
"Decide for yourself what success looks like when nobody's watching." – LNB

| HOW I FELT | 1 (DISSATISFIED) | 2 | 3 (SO-SO) | 4 | 5 (ON FIRE!) |
|---|---|---|---|---|---|
| MOOD | | | | | |
| ENERGY | | | | | |
| BLOOD SUGAR | | | | | |
| NUTRITION | | | | | |
| MINDSET | | | | | |

## TODAY I...

- ☐ EXERCISED
- ☐ MEDITATED
- ☐ EXPRESSED GRATITUDE
- ☐ SET GOALS FOR TODAY

- ☐ CHECKED MY SUGAR EVERY 2 HOURS
- ☐ WAS MINDFUL WHEN EATING
- ☐ MEAL PREPPED
- ☐ CARB COUNTED FOOD

- ☐ VISUALIZED DAY OF GOOD BLOOD SUGARS
- ☐ TOOK 10 DEEP BREATHS
- ☐ PRE-BOLUSED MEALS
- ☐ SPENT TIME WITH LOVED ONES

- ☐ TOOK A WALK OUTSIDE
- ☐ _____
- ☐ _____
- ☐ _____

EXERCISE: _____

WATER: ☐ ☐ ☐ ☐ ☐ ☐ ☐ ☐ ☐ ☐     TOTAL DAILY INSULIN: _____ UNITS

## THE NIGHT CAP

A PATTERN I RECOGNIZED WAS...

_____

_____

TOMORROW I WANT TO FOCUS MORE ON...

_____

_____

TODAY I CELEBRATE MYSELF BECAUSE...

_____

_____

# MORNING WORK IN

DATE: _____  S / M / T / W / T / F / S

## MINDSET PREP

I AM... _____

ONE THING I'M GRATEFUL FOR IS...

_____

ONE THING I DIDN'T DO YESTERDAY, BUT I WILL DO TODAY...

_____

## DAILY LOG

| TIME | BLOOD SUGAR | OUT OF RANGE (x) | INSULIN | C / F / P | NOTES / FOOD |
|------|-------------|------------------|---------|-----------|--------------|
|      |             |                  |         |           |              |
|      |             |                  |         |           |              |
|      |             |                  |         |           |              |
|      |             |                  |         |           |              |
|      |             |                  |         |           |              |
|      |             |                  |         |           |              |
|      |             |                  |         |           |              |
|      |             |                  |         |           |              |
|      |             |                  |         |           |              |
|      |             |                  |         |           |              |

# EVENING REFLECTION | "What doesn't kill you makes you stronger." – Friedrich Nietzsche

| HOW I FELT | 1 (DISSATISFIED) | 2 | 3 (SO-SO) | 4 | 5 (ON FIRE!) |
|---|---|---|---|---|---|
| MOOD | | | | | |
| ENERGY | | | | | |
| BLOOD SUGAR | | | | | |
| NUTRITION | | | | | |
| MINDSET | | | | | |

## TODAY I...

☐ EXERCISED    ☐ CHECKED MY SUGAR EVERY 2 HOURS    ☐ VISUALIZED DAY OF GOOD BLOOD SUGARS    ☐ TOOK A WALK OUTSIDE

☐ MEDITATED    ☐ WAS MINDFUL WHEN EATING    ☐ TOOK 10 DEEP BREATHS    ☐ _____

☐ EXPRESSED GRATITUDE    ☐ MEAL PREPPED    ☐ PRE-BOLUSED MEALS    ☐ _____

☐ SET GOALS FOR TODAY    ☐ CARB COUNTED FOOD    ☐ SPENT TIME WITH LOVED ONES    ☐ _____

EXERCISE: _____

WATER: ☐ ☐ ☐ ☐ ☐ ☐ ☐ ☐ ☐ ☐    TOTAL DAILY INSULIN: _____ UNITS

## THE NIGHT CAP

A PATTERN I RECOGNIZED WAS...

_____

_____

TOMORROW I WANT TO FOCUS MORE ON...

_____

_____

TODAY I CELEBRATE MYSELF BECAUSE...

_____

_____

# MORNING WORK IN

DATE: _____    S / M / T / W / T / F / S

I AM... _____

ONE THING I'M GRATEFUL FOR IS...

_____

ONE THING I DIDN'T DO YESTERDAY, BUT I WILL DO TODAY...

_____

## DAILY LOG

| TIME | BLOOD SUGAR | OUT OF RANGE (x) | INSULIN | C / F / P | NOTES / FOOD |
|------|-------------|------------------|---------|-----------|--------------|
|      |             |                  |         |           |              |
|      |             |                  |         |           |              |
|      |             |                  |         |           |              |
|      |             |                  |         |           |              |
|      |             |                  |         |           |              |
|      |             |                  |         |           |              |
|      |             |                  |         |           |              |
|      |             |                  |         |           |              |
|      |             |                  |         |           |              |
|      |             |                  |         |           |              |

# EVENING REFLECTION

"If something is wrong, fix it if you can. But train yourself not to worry. Worry never fixes anything." – Ernest Hemingway

| HOW I FELT | 1 (DISSATISFIED) | 2 | 3 (SO-SO) | 4 | 5 (ON FIRE!) |
|---|---|---|---|---|---|
| MOOD | | | | | |
| ENERGY | | | | | |
| BLOOD SUGAR | | | | | |
| NUTRITION | | | | | |
| MINDSET | | | | | |

## TODAY I...

- ☐ EXERCISED
- ☐ CHECKED MY SUGAR EVERY 2 HOURS
- ☐ VISUALIZED DAY OF GOOD BLOOD SUGARS
- ☐ TOOK A WALK OUTSIDE
- ☐ MEDITATED
- ☐ WAS MINDFUL WHEN EATING
- ☐ TOOK 10 DEEP BREATHS
- ☐ _____
- ☐ EXPRESSED GRATITUDE
- ☐ MEAL PREPPED
- ☐ PRE-BOLUSED MEALS
- ☐ _____
- ☐ SET GOALS FOR TODAY
- ☐ CARB COUNTED FOOD
- ☐ SPENT TIME WITH LOVED ONES
- ☐ _____

EXERCISE: _____

WATER: ☐ ☐ ☐ ☐ ☐ ☐ ☐ ☐ ☐ ☐     TOTAL DAILY INSULIN: _____ UNITS

## THE NIGHT CAP

A PATTERN I RECOGNIZED WAS...

_____
_____

TOMORROW I WANT TO FOCUS MORE ON...

_____
_____

TODAY I CELEBRATE MYSELF BECAUSE...

_____
_____

# MORNING WORK IN | DATE: _____ S / M / T / W / T / F / S

## MINDSET PREP

I AM... _____

ONE THING I'M GRATEFUL FOR IS...

_____

ONE THING I DIDN'T DO YESTERDAY, BUT I WILL DO TODAY...

_____

## DAILY LOG

| TIME | BLOOD SUGAR | OUT OF RANGE (x) | INSULIN | C / F / P | NOTES / FOOD |
|------|-------------|------------------|---------|-----------|--------------|
|      |             |                  |         |           |              |
|      |             |                  |         |           |              |
|      |             |                  |         |           |              |
|      |             |                  |         |           |              |
|      |             |                  |         |           |              |
|      |             |                  |         |           |              |
|      |             |                  |         |           |              |
|      |             |                  |         |           |              |
|      |             |                  |         |           |              |
|      |             |                  |         |           |              |

# EVENING REFLECTION | *I am greater than my highs and my lows.*

| HOW I FELT | 1 (DISSATISFIED) | 2 | 3 (SO-SO) | 4 | 5 (ON FIRE!) |
|---|---|---|---|---|---|
| MOOD | | | | | |
| ENERGY | | | | | |
| BLOOD SUGAR | | | | | |
| NUTRITION | | | | | |
| MINDSET | | | | | |

## TODAY I...

- ☐ EXERCISED
- ☐ MEDITATED
- ☐ EXPRESSED GRATITUDE
- ☐ SET GOALS FOR TODAY

- ☐ CHECKED MY SUGAR EVERY 2 HOURS
- ☐ WAS MINDFUL WHEN EATING
- ☐ MEAL PREPPED
- ☐ CARB COUNTED FOOD

- ☐ VISUALIZED DAY OF GOOD BLOOD SUGARS
- ☐ TOOK 10 DEEP BREATHS
- ☐ PRE-BOLUSED MEALS
- ☐ SPENT TIME WITH LOVED ONES

- ☐ TOOK A WALK OUTSIDE
- ☐ _____
- ☐ _____
- ☐ _____

EXERCISE: _____

WATER: 🥛🥛🥛🥛🥛🥛🥛🥛🥛🥛    TOTAL DAILY INSULIN: _____ UNITS

## THE NIGHT CAP

A PATTERN I RECOGNIZED WAS...

_____

_____

TOMORROW I WANT TO FOCUS MORE ON...

_____

_____

TODAY I CELEBRATE MYSELF BECAUSE...

_____

_____

# MORNING WORK IN | DATE: _____ S / M / T / W / T / F / S

I AM... _____

ONE THING I'M GRATEFUL FOR IS...

_____

ONE THING I DIDN'T DO YESTERDAY, BUT I WILL DO TODAY...

_____

## DAILY LOG

| TIME | BLOOD SUGAR | OUT OF RANGE (x) | INSULIN | C / F / P | NOTES / FOOD |
|------|------------|------------------|---------|-----------|--------------|
|      |            |                  |         |           |              |
|      |            |                  |         |           |              |
|      |            |                  |         |           |              |
|      |            |                  |         |           |              |
|      |            |                  |         |           |              |
|      |            |                  |         |           |              |
|      |            |                  |         |           |              |
|      |            |                  |         |           |              |
|      |            |                  |         |           |              |
|      |            |                  |         |           |              |

# EVENING REFLECTION

"The way we do anything is the way we do everything."
– Martha Beck

| HOW I FELT | 1<br>(DISSATISFIED) | 2 | 3<br>(SO-SO) | 4 | 5<br>(ON FIRE!) |
|---|---|---|---|---|---|
| MOOD | | | | | |
| ENERGY | | | | | |
| BLOOD SUGAR | | | | | |
| NUTRITION | | | | | |
| MINDSET | | | | | |

## TODAY I...

- [ ] EXERCISED
- [ ] MEDITATED
- [ ] EXPRESSED GRATITUDE
- [ ] SET GOALS FOR TODAY

- [ ] CHECKED MY SUGAR EVERY 2 HOURS
- [ ] WAS MINDFUL WHEN EATING
- [ ] MEAL PREPPED
- [ ] CARB COUNTED FOOD

- [ ] VISUALIZED DAY OF GOOD BLOOD SUGARS
- [ ] TOOK 10 DEEP BREATHS
- [ ] PRE-BOLUSED MEALS
- [ ] SPENT TIME WITH LOVED ONES

- [ ] TOOK A WALK OUTSIDE
- [ ] _____
- [ ] _____
- [ ] _____

EXERCISE: _____

WATER: ☐ ☐ ☐ ☐ ☐ ☐ ☐ ☐ ☐ ☐     TOTAL DAILY INSULIN: _____ UNITS

## THE NIGHT CAP

A PATTERN I RECOGNIZED WAS...

_____

_____

TOMORROW I WANT TO FOCUS MORE ON...

_____

_____

TODAY I CELEBRATE MYSELF BECAUSE...

_____

_____

# MORNING WORK IN | DATE: _____ S / M / T / W / T / F / S

## MINDSET PREP

I AM... _____

ONE THING I'M GRATEFUL FOR IS...

_____

ONE THING I DIDN'T DO YESTERDAY, BUT I WILL DO TODAY...

_____

## DAILY LOG

| TIME | BLOOD SUGAR | OUT OF RANGE (x) | INSULIN | C / F / P | NOTES / FOOD |
|------|-------------|------------------|---------|-----------|--------------|
|      |             |                  |         |           |              |
|      |             |                  |         |           |              |
|      |             |                  |         |           |              |
|      |             |                  |         |           |              |
|      |             |                  |         |           |              |
|      |             |                  |         |           |              |
|      |             |                  |         |           |              |
|      |             |                  |         |           |              |
|      |             |                  |         |           |              |
|      |             |                  |         |           |              |

# EVENING REFLECTION

**JOURNAL PROMPT:**
What is one thing you will forgive yourself for?

| HOW I FELT | 1 (DISSATISFIED) | 2 | 3 (SO-SO) | 4 | 5 (ON FIRE!) |
|---|---|---|---|---|---|
| MOOD | | | | | |
| ENERGY | | | | | |
| BLOOD SUGAR | | | | | |
| NUTRITION | | | | | |
| MINDSET | | | | | |

## TODAY I...

☐ EXERCISED    ☐ CHECKED MY SUGAR EVERY 2 HOURS    ☐ VISUALIZED DAY OF GOOD BLOOD SUGARS    ☐ TOOK A WALK OUTSIDE

☐ MEDITATED    ☐ WAS MINDFUL WHEN EATING    ☐ TOOK 10 DEEP BREATHS    ☐ _____

☐ EXPRESSED GRATITUDE    ☐ MEAL PREPPED    ☐ PRE-BOLUSED MEALS    ☐ _____

☐ SET GOALS FOR TODAY    ☐ CARB COUNTED FOOD    ☐ SPENT TIME WITH LOVED ONES    ☐ _____

EXERCISE: _____

WATER: ▽ ▽ ▽ ▽ ▽ ▽ ▽ ▽ ▽ ▽      TOTAL DAILY INSULIN: _____ UNITS

## THE NIGHT CAP

A PATTERN I RECOGNIZED WAS...

_____

_____

TOMORROW I WANT TO FOCUS MORE ON...

_____

_____

TODAY I CELEBRATE MYSELF BECAUSE...

_____

_____

# MORNING WORK IN | DATE: _____ S / M / T / W / T / F / S

## MINDSET PREP

I AM... _____

ONE THING I'M GRATEFUL FOR IS...

_____

ONE THING I DIDN'T DO YESTERDAY, BUT I WILL DO TODAY...

_____

## DAILY LOG

| TIME | BLOOD SUGAR | OUT OF RANGE (x) | INSULIN | C / F / P | NOTES / FOOD |
|------|-------------|------------------|---------|-----------|--------------|
|      |             |                  |         |           |              |
|      |             |                  |         |           |              |
|      |             |                  |         |           |              |
|      |             |                  |         |           |              |
|      |             |                  |         |           |              |
|      |             |                  |         |           |              |
|      |             |                  |         |           |              |
|      |             |                  |         |           |              |
|      |             |                  |         |           |              |
|      |             |                  |         |           |              |

# EVENING REFLECTION

"Others see you, the way you see you. All interactions are the sum of the love, kindness, patience, and honor you give yourself."
– LNB

| HOW I FELT | 1 (DISSATISFIED) | 2 | 3 (SO-SO) | 4 | 5 (ON FIRE!) |
|---|---|---|---|---|---|
| MOOD | | | | | |
| ENERGY | | | | | |
| BLOOD SUGAR | | | | | |
| NUTRITION | | | | | |
| MINDSET | | | | | |

## TODAY I...

- ☐ EXERCISED
- ☐ MEDITATED
- ☐ EXPRESSED GRATITUDE
- ☐ SET GOALS FOR TODAY

- ☐ CHECKED MY SUGAR EVERY 2 HOURS
- ☐ WAS MINDFUL WHEN EATING
- ☐ MEAL PREPPED
- ☐ CARB COUNTED FOOD

- ☐ VISUALIZED DAY OF GOOD BLOOD SUGARS
- ☐ TOOK 10 DEEP BREATHS
- ☐ PRE-BOLUSED MEALS
- ☐ SPENT TIME WITH LOVED ONES

- ☐ TOOK A WALK OUTSIDE
- ☐ _____
- ☐ _____
- ☐ _____

EXERCISE: _____

WATER: ☐ ☐ ☐ ☐ ☐ ☐ ☐ ☐ ☐ ☐     TOTAL DAILY INSULIN: _____ UNITS

## THE NIGHT CAP

A PATTERN I RECOGNIZED WAS...

_____

_____

TOMORROW I WANT TO FOCUS MORE ON...

_____

_____

TODAY I CELEBRATE MYSELF BECAUSE...

_____

_____

# MORNING WORK IN | DATE: _____ S / M / T / W / T / F / S

## MINDSET PREP

I AM... _____

ONE THING I'M GRATEFUL FOR IS...

_____

ONE THING I DIDN'T DO YESTERDAY, BUT I WILL DO TODAY...

_____

## DAILY LOG

| TIME | BLOOD SUGAR | OUT OF RANGE (x) | INSULIN | C / F / P | NOTES / FOOD |
|------|-------------|------------------|---------|-----------|--------------|
|      |             |                  |         |           |              |
|      |             |                  |         |           |              |
|      |             |                  |         |           |              |
|      |             |                  |         |           |              |
|      |             |                  |         |           |              |
|      |             |                  |         |           |              |
|      |             |                  |         |           |              |
|      |             |                  |         |           |              |
|      |             |                  |         |           |              |
|      |             |                  |         |           |              |

# EVENING REFLECTION | "You don't have to have it all figured out to move forward."
– Roy T. Bennett

## HOW I FELT

| | 1 (DISSATISFIED) | 2 | 3 (SO-SO) | 4 | 5 (ON FIRE!) |
|---|---|---|---|---|---|
| MOOD | | | | | |
| ENERGY | | | | | |
| BLOOD SUGAR | | | | | |
| NUTRITION | | | | | |
| MINDSET | | | | | |

## TODAY I...

☐ EXERCISED

☐ MEDITATED

☐ EXPRESSED GRATITUDE

☐ SET GOALS FOR TODAY

☐ CHECKED MY SUGAR EVERY 2 HOURS

☐ WAS MINDFUL WHEN EATING

☐ MEAL PREPPED

☐ CARB COUNTED FOOD

☐ VISUALIZED DAY OF GOOD BLOOD SUGARS

☐ TOOK 10 DEEP BREATHS

☐ PRE-BOLUSED MEALS

☐ SPENT TIME WITH LOVED ONES

☐ TOOK A WALK OUTSIDE

☐ _____

☐ _____

☐ _____

EXERCISE: _____

WATER: ☐ ☐ ☐ ☐ ☐ ☐ ☐ ☐ ☐ ☐          TOTAL DAILY INSULIN: _____ UNITS

## THE NIGHT CAP

A PATTERN I RECOGNIZED WAS...

_____

_____

TOMORROW I WANT TO FOCUS MORE ON...

_____

_____

TODAY I CELEBRATE MYSELF BECAUSE...

_____

_____

# MORNING WORK IN | DATE: _____ S / M / T / W / T / F / S

## MINDSET PREP | I AM... _____

ONE THING I'M GRATEFUL FOR IS...

_____

ONE THING I DIDN'T DO YESTERDAY, BUT I WILL DO TODAY...

_____

## DAILY LOG

| TIME | BLOOD SUGAR | OUT OF RANGE (x) | INSULIN | C / F / P | NOTES / FOOD |
|------|-------------|------------------|---------|-----------|--------------|
|      |             |                  |         |           |              |
|      |             |                  |         |           |              |
|      |             |                  |         |           |              |
|      |             |                  |         |           |              |
|      |             |                  |         |           |              |
|      |             |                  |         |           |              |
|      |             |                  |         |           |              |
|      |             |                  |         |           |              |
|      |             |                  |         |           |              |
|      |             |                  |         |           |              |

# EVENING REFLECTION | "Mindfulness is a way of befriending ourselves and our experience." – Jon Kabat-Zinn

## HOW I FELT

| | 1 (DISSATISFIED) | 2 | 3 (SO-SO) | 4 | 5 (ON FIRE!) |
|---|---|---|---|---|---|
| MOOD | | | | | |
| ENERGY | | | | | |
| BLOOD SUGAR | | | | | |
| NUTRITION | | | | | |
| MINDSET | | | | | |

## TODAY I...

☐ EXERCISED        ☐ CHECKED MY SUGAR EVERY 2 HOURS        ☐ VISUALIZED DAY OF GOOD BLOOD SUGARS        ☐ TOOK A WALK OUTSIDE

☐ MEDITATED        ☐ WAS MINDFUL WHEN EATING        ☐ TOOK 10 DEEP BREATHS        ☐ _____

☐ EXPRESSED GRATITUDE        ☐ MEAL PREPPED        ☐ PRE-BOLUSED MEALS        ☐ _____

☐ SET GOALS FOR TODAY        ☐ CARB COUNTED FOOD        ☐ SPENT TIME WITH LOVED ONES        ☐ _____

EXERCISE: _____

WATER: ▽ ▽ ▽ ▽ ▽ ▽ ▽ ▽ ▽ ▽        TOTAL DAILY INSULIN: _____ UNITS

## THE NIGHT CAP

A PATTERN I RECOGNIZED WAS...

_____

_____

TOMORROW I WANT TO FOCUS MORE ON...

_____

_____

TODAY I CELEBRATE MYSELF BECAUSE...

_____

_____

# MORNING WORK IN | DATE: _____ S / M / T / W / T / F / S

## MINDSET PREP

I AM... _____

ONE THING I'M GRATEFUL FOR IS...

_____

ONE THING I DIDN'T DO YESTERDAY, BUT I WILL DO TODAY...

_____

## DAILY LOG

| TIME | BLOOD SUGAR | OUT OF RANGE (x) | INSULIN | C / F / P | NOTES / FOOD |
|------|-------------|------------------|---------|-----------|--------------|
|      |             |                  |         |           |              |
|      |             |                  |         |           |              |
|      |             |                  |         |           |              |
|      |             |                  |         |           |              |
|      |             |                  |         |           |              |
|      |             |                  |         |           |              |
|      |             |                  |         |           |              |
|      |             |                  |         |           |              |
|      |             |                  |         |           |              |

# EVENING REFLECTION | "Vulnerability is not weakness." – Brené Brown

| HOW I FELT | 1 (DISSATISFIED) | 2 | 3 (SO-SO) | 4 | 5 (ON FIRE!) |
|---|---|---|---|---|---|
| MOOD | | | | | |
| ENERGY | | | | | |
| BLOOD SUGAR | | | | | |
| NUTRITION | | | | | |
| MINDSET | | | | | |

## TODAY I...

- ☐ EXERCISED
- ☐ MEDITATED
- ☐ EXPRESSED GRATITUDE
- ☐ SET GOALS FOR TODAY

- ☐ CHECKED MY SUGAR EVERY 2 HOURS
- ☐ WAS MINDFUL WHEN EATING
- ☐ MEAL PREPPED
- ☐ CARB COUNTED FOOD

- ☐ VISUALIZED DAY OF GOOD BLOOD SUGARS
- ☐ TOOK 10 DEEP BREATHS
- ☐ PRE-BOLUSED MEALS
- ☐ SPENT TIME WITH LOVED ONES

- ☐ TOOK A WALK OUTSIDE
- ☐ _____
- ☐ _____
- ☐ _____

EXERCISE: _____

WATER: ☐ ☐ ☐ ☐ ☐ ☐ ☐ ☐ ☐ ☐     TOTAL DAILY INSULIN: _____ UNITS

## THE NIGHT CAP

A PATTERN I RECOGNIZED WAS...

_____

_____

TOMORROW I WANT TO FOCUS MORE ON...

_____

_____

TODAY I CELEBRATE MYSELF BECAUSE...

_____

_____

# MORNING WORK IN

## MINDSET PREP

I AM... _____

ONE THING I'M GRATEFUL FOR IS...

_____

ONE THING I DIDN'T DO YESTERDAY, BUT I WILL DO TODAY...

_____

## DAILY LOG

| TIME | BLOOD SUGAR | OUT OF RANGE (x) | INSULIN | C / F / P | NOTES / FOOD |
|------|-------------|------------------|---------|-----------|--------------|
|      |             |                  |         |           |              |
|      |             |                  |         |           |              |
|      |             |                  |         |           |              |
|      |             |                  |         |           |              |
|      |             |                  |         |           |              |
|      |             |                  |         |           |              |
|      |             |                  |         |           |              |
|      |             |                  |         |           |              |
|      |             |                  |         |           |              |
|      |             |                  |         |           |              |

# EVENING REFLECTION | *Don't look backwards, you're not going that way.*

| HOW I FELT | 1 (DISSATISFIED) | 2 | 3 (SO-SO) | 4 | 5 (ON FIRE!) |
|---|---|---|---|---|---|
| MOOD | | | | | |
| ENERGY | | | | | |
| BLOOD SUGAR | | | | | |
| NUTRITION | | | | | |
| MINDSET | | | | | |

## TODAY I...

- ☐ EXERCISED
- ☐ CHECKED MY SUGAR EVERY 2 HOURS
- ☐ VISUALIZED DAY OF GOOD BLOOD SUGARS
- ☐ TOOK A WALK OUTSIDE

- ☐ MEDITATED
- ☐ WAS MINDFUL WHEN EATING
- ☐ TOOK 10 DEEP BREATHS
- ☐ _____

- ☐ EXPRESSED GRATITUDE
- ☐ MEAL PREPPED
- ☐ PRE-BOLUSED MEALS
- ☐ _____

- ☐ SET GOALS FOR TODAY
- ☐ CARB COUNTED FOOD
- ☐ SPENT TIME WITH LOVED ONES
- ☐ _____

EXERCISE: _____

WATER: ⬜ ⬜ ⬜ ⬜ ⬜ ⬜ ⬜ ⬜ ⬜ ⬜      TOTAL DAILY INSULIN: _____ UNITS

## THE NIGHT CAP

A PATTERN I RECOGNIZED WAS...

_____

_____

TOMORROW I WANT TO FOCUS MORE ON...

_____

_____

TODAY I CELEBRATE MYSELF BECAUSE...

_____

_____

# MORNING WORK IN

DATE: _____

## MINDSET PREP

I AM... _____

ONE THING I'M GRATEFUL FOR IS...

_____

ONE THING I DIDN'T DO YESTERDAY, BUT I WILL DO TODAY...

_____

## DAILY LOG

| TIME | BLOOD SUGAR | OUT OF RANGE (x) | INSULIN | C / F / P | NOTES / FOOD |
|------|-------------|------------------|---------|-----------|--------------|
|      |             |                  |         |           |              |
|      |             |                  |         |           |              |
|      |             |                  |         |           |              |
|      |             |                  |         |           |              |
|      |             |                  |         |           |              |
|      |             |                  |         |           |              |
|      |             |                  |         |           |              |
|      |             |                  |         |           |              |
|      |             |                  |         |           |              |
|      |             |                  |         |           |              |

# EVENING REFLECTION

**JOURNAL PROMPT:**
How can you love yourself a little extra today?

| HOW I FELT | 1<br>(DISSATISFIED) | 2 | 3<br>(SO-SO) | 4 | 5<br>(ON FIRE!) |
|---|---|---|---|---|---|
| MOOD | | | | | |
| ENERGY | | | | | |
| BLOOD SUGAR | | | | | |
| NUTRITION | | | | | |
| MINDSET | | | | | |

## TODAY I...

- [ ] EXERCISED
- [ ] MEDITATED
- [ ] EXPRESSED GRATITUDE
- [ ] SET GOALS FOR TODAY

- [ ] CHECKED MY SUGAR EVERY 2 HOURS
- [ ] WAS MINDFUL WHEN EATING
- [ ] MEAL PREPPED
- [ ] CARB COUNTED FOOD

- [ ] VISUALIZED DAY OF GOOD BLOOD SUGARS
- [ ] TOOK 10 DEEP BREATHS
- [ ] PRE-BOLUSED MEALS
- [ ] SPENT TIME WITH LOVED ONES

- [ ] TOOK A WALK OUTSIDE
- [ ] _____
- [ ] _____
- [ ] _____

EXERCISE: _____

WATER: ⊽ ⊽ ⊽ ⊽ ⊽ ⊽ ⊽ ⊽ ⊽ ⊽        TOTAL DAILY INSULIN: _____ UNITS

## THE NIGHT CAP

A PATTERN I RECOGNIZED WAS...

_____

_____

TOMORROW I WANT TO FOCUS MORE ON...

_____

_____

TODAY I CELEBRATE MYSELF BECAUSE...

_____

_____

# MORNING WORK IN

DATE: _____

## MINDSET PREP

I AM... _____

ONE THING I'M GRATEFUL FOR IS...

_____

ONE THING I DIDN'T DO YESTERDAY, BUT I WILL DO TODAY...

_____

## DAILY LOG

| TIME | BLOOD SUGAR | OUT OF RANGE (x) | INSULIN | C / F / P | NOTES / FOOD |
|------|-------------|------------------|---------|-----------|--------------|
|      |             |                  |         |           |              |
|      |             |                  |         |           |              |
|      |             |                  |         |           |              |
|      |             |                  |         |           |              |
|      |             |                  |         |           |              |
|      |             |                  |         |           |              |
|      |             |                  |         |           |              |
|      |             |                  |         |           |              |
|      |             |                  |         |           |              |
|      |             |                  |         |           |              |

# EVENING REFLECTION
"Adopt the pace of nature, her secret is patience."
– Ralph Waldo Emerson

| HOW I FELT | 1 (DISSATISFIED) | 2 | 3 (SO-SO) | 4 | 5 (ON FIRE!) |
|---|---|---|---|---|---|
| MOOD | | | | | |
| ENERGY | | | | | |
| BLOOD SUGAR | | | | | |
| NUTRITION | | | | | |
| MINDSET | | | | | |

## TODAY I...

- ☐ EXERCISED
- ☐ CHECKED MY SUGAR EVERY 2 HOURS
- ☐ VISUALIZED DAY OF GOOD BLOOD SUGARS
- ☐ TOOK A WALK OUTSIDE

- ☐ MEDITATED
- ☐ WAS MINDFUL WHEN EATING
- ☐ TOOK 10 DEEP BREATHS
- ☐ _____

- ☐ EXPRESSED GRATITUDE
- ☐ MEAL PREPPED
- ☐ PRE-BOLUSED MEALS
- ☐ _____

- ☐ SET GOALS FOR TODAY
- ☐ CARB COUNTED FOOD
- ☐ SPENT TIME WITH LOVED ONES
- ☐ _____

EXERCISE: _____

WATER: ☐ ☐ ☐ ☐ ☐ ☐ ☐ ☐ ☐ ☐        TOTAL DAILY INSULIN: _____ UNITS

## THE NIGHT CAP

A PATTERN I RECOGNIZED WAS...

_____
_____

TOMORROW I WANT TO FOCUS MORE ON...

_____
_____

TODAY I CELEBRATE MYSELF BECAUSE...

_____
_____

# MORNING WORK IN

DATE: _____

S / M / T / W / T / F / S

## MINDSET PREP

I AM... _____

ONE THING I'M GRATEFUL FOR IS...

_____

ONE THING I DIDN'T DO YESTERDAY, BUT I WILL DO TODAY...

_____

## DAILY LOG

| TIME | BLOOD SUGAR | OUT OF RANGE (X) | INSULIN | C / F / P | NOTES / FOOD |
|------|-------------|------------------|---------|-----------|--------------|
|      |             |                  |         |           |              |
|      |             |                  |         |           |              |
|      |             |                  |         |           |              |
|      |             |                  |         |           |              |
|      |             |                  |         |           |              |
|      |             |                  |         |           |              |
|      |             |                  |         |           |              |
|      |             |                  |         |           |              |
|      |             |                  |         |           |              |
|      |             |                  |         |           |              |

# EVENING REFLECTION

"The things that matter most in our lives are not fantastic or grand. They are moments when we touch one another."
– Jack Kornfield

| HOW I FELT | 1 (DISSATISFIED) | 2 | 3 (SO-SO) | 4 | 5 (ON FIRE!) |
|---|---|---|---|---|---|
| MOOD | | | | | |
| ENERGY | | | | | |
| BLOOD SUGAR | | | | | |
| NUTRITION | | | | | |
| MINDSET | | | | | |

## TODAY I...

- ☐ EXERCISED
- ☐ MEDITATED
- ☐ EXPRESSED GRATITUDE
- ☐ SET GOALS FOR TODAY

- ☐ CHECKED MY SUGAR EVERY 2 HOURS
- ☐ WAS MINDFUL WHEN EATING
- ☐ MEAL PREPPED
- ☐ CARB COUNTED FOOD

- ☐ VISUALIZED DAY OF GOOD BLOOD SUGARS
- ☐ TOOK 10 DEEP BREATHS
- ☐ PRE-BOLUSED MEALS
- ☐ SPENT TIME WITH LOVED ONES

- ☐ TOOK A WALK OUTSIDE
- ☐ _____
- ☐ _____
- ☐ _____

EXERCISE: _____

WATER: ☐ ☐ ☐ ☐ ☐ ☐ ☐ ☐ ☐ ☐     TOTAL DAILY INSULIN: _____ UNITS

## THE NIGHT CAP

A PATTERN I RECOGNIZED WAS...

_____

_____

TOMORROW I WANT TO FOCUS MORE ON...

_____

_____

TODAY I CELEBRATE MYSELF BECAUSE...

_____

_____

# MORNING WORK IN | DATE: _____ S / M / T / W / T / F / S

## MINDSET PREP

I AM... _____

ONE THING I'M GRATEFUL FOR IS...

_____

ONE THING I DIDN'T DO YESTERDAY, BUT I WILL DO TODAY...

_____

## DAILY LOG

| TIME | BLOOD SUGAR | OUT OF RANGE (x) | INSULIN | C / F / P | NOTES / FOOD |
|------|-------------|------------------|---------|-----------|--------------|
|      |             |                  |         |           |              |
|      |             |                  |         |           |              |
|      |             |                  |         |           |              |
|      |             |                  |         |           |              |
|      |             |                  |         |           |              |
|      |             |                  |         |           |              |
|      |             |                  |         |           |              |
|      |             |                  |         |           |              |
|      |             |                  |         |           |              |

# EVENING REFLECTION | "Live each day as commander in chief of your life." – LNB

| HOW I FELT | 1 (DISSATISFIED) | 2 | 3 (SO-SO) | 4 | 5 (ON FIRE!) |
|---|---|---|---|---|---|
| MOOD | | | | | |
| ENERGY | | | | | |
| BLOOD SUGAR | | | | | |
| NUTRITION | | | | | |
| MINDSET | | | | | |

## TODAY I...

- ☐ EXERCISED
- ☐ CHECKED MY SUGAR EVERY 2 HOURS
- ☐ VISUALIZED DAY OF GOOD BLOOD SUGARS
- ☐ TOOK A WALK OUTSIDE

- ☐ MEDITATED
- ☐ WAS MINDFUL WHEN EATING
- ☐ TOOK 10 DEEP BREATHS
- ☐ _____

- ☐ EXPRESSED GRATITUDE
- ☐ MEAL PREPPED
- ☐ PRE-BOLUSED MEALS
- ☐ _____

- ☐ SET GOALS FOR TODAY
- ☐ CARB COUNTED FOOD
- ☐ SPENT TIME WITH LOVED ONES
- ☐ _____

EXERCISE: _____

WATER: ▽ ▽ ▽ ▽ ▽ ▽ ▽ ▽ ▽ ▽          TOTAL DAILY INSULIN: _____ UNITS

## THE NIGHT CAP

A PATTERN I RECOGNIZED WAS...

_____

_____

TOMORROW I WANT TO FOCUS MORE ON...

_____

_____

TODAY I CELEBRATE MYSELF BECAUSE...

_____

_____

# MORNING WORK IN | DATE: _____ S / M / T / W / T / F / S

## MINDSET PREP

I AM... _____

ONE THING I'M GRATEFUL FOR IS...

_____

ONE THING I DIDN'T DO YESTERDAY, BUT I WILL DO TODAY...

_____

## DAILY LOG

| TIME | BLOOD SUGAR | OUT OF RANGE (x) | INSULIN | C / F / P | NOTES / FOOD |
|------|-------------|------------------|---------|-----------|--------------|
|      |             |                  |         |           |              |
|      |             |                  |         |           |              |
|      |             |                  |         |           |              |
|      |             |                  |         |           |              |
|      |             |                  |         |           |              |
|      |             |                  |         |           |              |
|      |             |                  |         |           |              |
|      |             |                  |         |           |              |
|      |             |                  |         |           |              |
|      |             |                  |         |           |              |

# EVENING REFLECTION | "Control the controllable. Release the rest." – Patrick Rohe

| HOW I FELT | 1 (DISSATISFIED) | 2 | 3 (SO-SO) | 4 | 5 (ON FIRE!) |
|---|---|---|---|---|---|
| MOOD | | | | | |
| ENERGY | | | | | |
| BLOOD SUGAR | | | | | |
| NUTRITION | | | | | |
| MINDSET | | | | | |

## TODAY I...

- ☐ EXERCISED
- ☐ MEDITATED
- ☐ EXPRESSED GRATITUDE
- ☐ SET GOALS FOR TODAY

- ☐ CHECKED MY SUGAR EVERY 2 HOURS
- ☐ WAS MINDFUL WHEN EATING
- ☐ MEAL PREPPED
- ☐ CARB COUNTED FOOD

- ☐ VISUALIZED DAY OF GOOD BLOOD SUGARS
- ☐ TOOK 10 DEEP BREATHS
- ☐ PRE-BOLUSED MEALS
- ☐ SPENT TIME WITH LOVED ONES

- ☐ TOOK A WALK OUTSIDE
- ☐ _____
- ☐ _____
- ☐ _____

EXERCISE: _____

WATER: ☐ ☐ ☐ ☐ ☐ ☐ ☐ ☐ ☐ ☐        TOTAL DAILY INSULIN: _____ UNITS

## THE NIGHT CAP

A PATTERN I RECOGNIZED WAS...

_____

_____

TOMORROW I WANT TO FOCUS MORE ON...

_____

_____

TODAY I CELEBRATE MYSELF BECAUSE...

_____

_____

# MORNING WORK IN | DATE: _____  S / M / T / W / T / F / S

## MINDSET PREP

I AM... _____

ONE THING I'M GRATEFUL FOR IS...

_____

ONE THING I DIDN'T DO YESTERDAY, BUT I WILL DO TODAY...

_____

## DAILY LOG

| TIME | BLOOD SUGAR | OUT OF RANGE (x) | INSULIN | C / F / P | NOTES / FOOD |
|------|-------------|------------------|---------|-----------|--------------|
|      |             |                  |         |           |              |
|      |             |                  |         |           |              |
|      |             |                  |         |           |              |
|      |             |                  |         |           |              |
|      |             |                  |         |           |              |
|      |             |                  |         |           |              |
|      |             |                  |         |           |              |
|      |             |                  |         |           |              |
|      |             |                  |         |           |              |
|      |             |                  |         |           |              |

# EVENING REFLECTION

"Fear is a natural reaction to moving closer to the truth."
– Pema Chödrön

| HOW I FELT | 1 (DISSATISFIED) | 2 | 3 (SO-SO) | 4 | 5 (ON FIRE!) |
|---|---|---|---|---|---|
| MOOD | | | | | |
| ENERGY | | | | | |
| BLOOD SUGAR | | | | | |
| NUTRITION | | | | | |
| MINDSET | | | | | |

## TODAY I...

- ☐ EXERCISED
- ☐ MEDITATED
- ☐ EXPRESSED GRATITUDE
- ☐ SET GOALS FOR TODAY

- ☐ CHECKED MY SUGAR EVERY 2 HOURS
- ☐ WAS MINDFUL WHEN EATING
- ☐ MEAL PREPPED
- ☐ CARB COUNTED FOOD

- ☐ VISUALIZED DAY OF GOOD BLOOD SUGARS
- ☐ TOOK 10 DEEP BREATHS
- ☐ PRE-BOLUSED MEALS
- ☐ SPENT TIME WITH LOVED ONES

- ☐ TOOK A WALK OUTSIDE
- ☐ _____
- ☐ _____
- ☐ _____

EXERCISE: _____

WATER: ☐ ☐ ☐ ☐ ☐ ☐ ☐ ☐ ☐ ☐     TOTAL DAILY INSULIN: _____ UNITS

## THE NIGHT CAP

A PATTERN I RECOGNIZED WAS...

_____

_____

TOMORROW I WANT TO FOCUS MORE ON...

_____

_____

TODAY I CELEBRATE MYSELF BECAUSE...

_____

_____

# MORNING WORK IN | DATE: _____ S / M / T / W / T / F / S

I AM... _____

ONE THING I'M GRATEFUL FOR IS...

_____

ONE THING I DIDN'T DO YESTERDAY, BUT I WILL DO TODAY...

_____

## DAILY LOG

| TIME | BLOOD SUGAR | OUT OF RANGE (x) | INSULIN | C / F / P | NOTES / FOOD |
|------|-------------|------------------|---------|-----------|--------------|
|      |             |                  |         |           |              |
|      |             |                  |         |           |              |
|      |             |                  |         |           |              |
|      |             |                  |         |           |              |
|      |             |                  |         |           |              |
|      |             |                  |         |           |              |
|      |             |                  |         |           |              |
|      |             |                  |         |           |              |
|      |             |                  |         |           |              |
|      |             |                  |         |           |              |

# EVENING REFLECTION | *Reset. Readjust. Restart. Refocus. As many times as you need to.*

| HOW I FELT | 1 (DISSATISFIED) | 2 | 3 (SO-SO) | 4 | 5 (ON FIRE!) |
|---|---|---|---|---|---|
| MOOD | | | | | |
| ENERGY | | | | | |
| BLOOD SUGAR | | | | | |
| NUTRITION | | | | | |
| MINDSET | | | | | |

## TODAY I...

☐ EXERCISED    ☐ CHECKED MY SUGAR EVERY 2 HOURS    ☐ VISUALIZED DAY OF GOOD BLOOD SUGARS    ☐ TOOK A WALK OUTSIDE

☐ MEDITATED    ☐ WAS MINDFUL WHEN EATING    ☐ TOOK 10 DEEP BREATHS    ☐ _____

☐ EXPRESSED GRATITUDE    ☐ MEAL PREPPED    ☐ PRE-BOLUSED MEALS    ☐ _____

☐ SET GOALS FOR TODAY    ☐ CARB COUNTED FOOD    ☐ SPENT TIME WITH LOVED ONES    ☐ _____

EXERCISE: _____

WATER: ☐ ☐ ☐ ☐ ☐ ☐ ☐ ☐ ☐ ☐     TOTAL DAILY INSULIN: _____ UNITS

## THE NIGHT CAP

A PATTERN I RECOGNIZED WAS...

_____

_____

TOMORROW I WANT TO FOCUS MORE ON...

_____

_____

TODAY I CELEBRATE MYSELF BECAUSE...

_____

_____

# MORNING WORK IN | DATE: _____  S / M / T / W / T / F / S

## MINDSET PREP

I AM... _____

ONE THING I'M GRATEFUL FOR IS...

_____

ONE THING I DIDN'T DO YESTERDAY, BUT I WILL DO TODAY...

_____

## DAILY LOG

| TIME | BLOOD SUGAR | OUT OF RANGE (x) | INSULIN | C / F / P | NOTES / FOOD |
|------|-------------|------------------|---------|-----------|--------------|
|      |             |                  |         |           |              |
|      |             |                  |         |           |              |
|      |             |                  |         |           |              |
|      |             |                  |         |           |              |
|      |             |                  |         |           |              |
|      |             |                  |         |           |              |
|      |             |                  |         |           |              |
|      |             |                  |         |           |              |
|      |             |                  |         |           |              |
|      |             |                  |         |           |              |

# EVENING REFLECTION

| HOW I FELT | 1 (DISSATISFIED) | 2 | 3 (SO-SO) | 4 | 5 (ON FIRE!) |
|---|---|---|---|---|---|
| MOOD | | | | | |
| ENERGY | | | | | |
| BLOOD SUGAR | | | | | |
| NUTRITION | | | | | |
| MINDSET | | | | | |

## TODAY I...

- [ ] EXERCISED
- [ ] MEDITATED
- [ ] EXPRESSED GRATITUDE
- [ ] SET GOALS FOR TODAY

- [ ] CHECKED MY SUGAR EVERY 2 HOURS
- [ ] WAS MINDFUL WHEN EATING
- [ ] MEAL PREPPED
- [ ] CARB COUNTED FOOD

- [ ] VISUALIZED DAY OF GOOD BLOOD SUGARS
- [ ] TOOK 10 DEEP BREATHS
- [ ] PRE-BOLUSED MEALS
- [ ] SPENT TIME WITH LOVED ONES

- [ ] TOOK A WALK OUTSIDE
- [ ] _____
- [ ] _____
- [ ] _____

EXERCISE: _____

WATER: 🥤 🥤 🥤 🥤 🥤 🥤 🥤 🥤 🥤 🥤          TOTAL DAILY INSULIN: _____ UNITS

## THE NIGHT CAP

A PATTERN I RECOGNIZED WAS...

_____

_____

TOMORROW I WANT TO FOCUS MORE ON...

_____

_____

TODAY I CELEBRATE MYSELF BECAUSE...

_____

_____

# MORNING WORK IN

DATE: _____     S / M / T / W / T / F / S

## MINDSET PREP

I AM... _____

ONE THING I'M GRATEFUL FOR IS...

_____

ONE THING I DIDN'T DO YESTERDAY, BUT I WILL DO TODAY...

_____

## DAILY LOG

| TIME | BLOOD SUGAR | OUT OF RANGE (x) | INSULIN | C / F / P | NOTES / FOOD |
|------|-------------|------------------|---------|-----------|--------------|
|      |             |                  |         |           |              |
|      |             |                  |         |           |              |
|      |             |                  |         |           |              |
|      |             |                  |         |           |              |
|      |             |                  |         |           |              |
|      |             |                  |         |           |              |
|      |             |                  |         |           |              |
|      |             |                  |         |           |              |
|      |             |                  |         |           |              |
|      |             |                  |         |           |              |

# EVENING REFLECTION

"It is our most challenging seasons that serve as our greatest teachers." – Danielle Doby

| HOW I FELT | 1 (DISSATISFIED) | 2 | 3 (SO-SO) | 4 | 5 (ON FIRE!) |
|---|---|---|---|---|---|
| MOOD | | | | | |
| ENERGY | | | | | |
| BLOOD SUGAR | | | | | |
| NUTRITION | | | | | |
| MINDSET | | | | | |

## TODAY I...

- ☐ EXERCISED
- ☐ CHECKED MY SUGAR EVERY 2 HOURS
- ☐ VISUALIZED DAY OF GOOD BLOOD SUGARS
- ☐ TOOK A WALK OUTSIDE

- ☐ MEDITATED
- ☐ WAS MINDFUL WHEN EATING
- ☐ TOOK 10 DEEP BREATHS
- ☐ _____

- ☐ EXPRESSED GRATITUDE
- ☐ MEAL PREPPED
- ☐ PRE-BOLUSED MEALS
- ☐ _____

- ☐ SET GOALS FOR TODAY
- ☐ CARB COUNTED FOOD
- ☐ SPENT TIME WITH LOVED ONES
- ☐ _____

EXERCISE: _____

WATER: ▽ ▽ ▽ ▽ ▽ ▽ ▽ ▽ ▽ ▽    TOTAL DAILY INSULIN: _____ UNITS

## THE NIGHT CAP

A PATTERN I RECOGNIZED WAS...

_____

_____

TOMORROW I WANT TO FOCUS MORE ON...

_____

_____

TODAY I CELEBRATE MYSELF BECAUSE...

_____

_____

# MORNING WORK IN | DATE: _____ S / M / T / W / T / F / S

## MINDSET PREP

I AM... _____

ONE THING I'M GRATEFUL FOR IS...

_____

ONE THING I DIDN'T DO YESTERDAY, BUT I WILL DO TODAY...

_____

## DAILY LOG

| TIME | BLOOD SUGAR | OUT OF RANGE (x) | INSULIN | C / F / P | NOTES / FOOD |
|------|-------------|------------------|---------|-----------|--------------|
|      |             |                  |         |           |              |
|      |             |                  |         |           |              |
|      |             |                  |         |           |              |
|      |             |                  |         |           |              |
|      |             |                  |         |           |              |
|      |             |                  |         |           |              |
|      |             |                  |         |           |              |
|      |             |                  |         |           |              |
|      |             |                  |         |           |              |
|      |             |                  |         |           |              |

# EVENING REFLECTION

| "The six best doctors: Sunshine, Water, Rest, Air, Exercise, and Diet." – Wayne Fields

| HOW I FELT | 1 (DISSATISFIED) | 2 | 3 (SO-SO) | 4 | 5 (ON FIRE!) |
|---|---|---|---|---|---|
| MOOD | | | | | |
| ENERGY | | | | | |
| BLOOD SUGAR | | | | | |
| NUTRITION | | | | | |
| MINDSET | | | | | |

## TODAY I...

- ☐ EXERCISED
- ☐ CHECKED MY SUGAR EVERY 2 HOURS
- ☐ VISUALIZED DAY OF GOOD BLOOD SUGARS
- ☐ TOOK A WALK OUTSIDE

- ☐ MEDITATED
- ☐ WAS MINDFUL WHEN EATING
- ☐ TOOK 10 DEEP BREATHS
- ☐ _____

- ☐ EXPRESSED GRATITUDE
- ☐ MEAL PREPPED
- ☐ PRE-BOLUSED MEALS
- ☐ _____

- ☐ SET GOALS FOR TODAY
- ☐ CARB COUNTED FOOD
- ☐ SPENT TIME WITH LOVED ONES
- ☐ _____

EXERCISE: _____

WATER: ▯ ▯ ▯ ▯ ▯ ▯ ▯ ▯ ▯ ▯     TOTAL DAILY INSULIN: _____ UNITS

## THE NIGHT CAP

A PATTERN I RECOGNIZED WAS...

_____

_____

TOMORROW I WANT TO FOCUS MORE ON...

_____

_____

TODAY I CELEBRATE MYSELF BECAUSE...

_____

_____

# MORNING WORK IN | DATE: _____

## MINDSET PREP

I AM... _____

ONE THING I'M GRATEFUL FOR IS...

_____

ONE THING I DIDN'T DO YESTERDAY, BUT I WILL DO TODAY...

_____

## DAILY LOG

| TIME | BLOOD SUGAR | OUT OF RANGE (x) | INSULIN | C / F / P | NOTES / FOOD |
|------|-------------|------------------|---------|-----------|--------------|
|      |             |                  |         |           |              |
|      |             |                  |         |           |              |
|      |             |                  |         |           |              |
|      |             |                  |         |           |              |
|      |             |                  |         |           |              |
|      |             |                  |         |           |              |
|      |             |                  |         |           |              |
|      |             |                  |         |           |              |
|      |             |                  |         |           |              |

# EVENING REFLECTION

| "The road to sustained happiness is about disciplining your behavior." – Will Smith

| HOW I FELT | 1 (DISSATISFIED) | 2 | 3 (SO-SO) | 4 | 5 (ON FIRE!) |
|---|---|---|---|---|---|
| MOOD | | | | | |
| ENERGY | | | | | |
| BLOOD SUGAR | | | | | |
| NUTRITION | | | | | |
| MINDSET | | | | | |

## TODAY I...

☐ EXERCISED ☐ CHECKED MY SUGAR EVERY 2 HOURS ☐ VISUALIZED DAY OF GOOD BLOOD SUGARS ☐ TOOK A WALK OUTSIDE

☐ MEDITATED ☐ WAS MINDFUL WHEN EATING ☐ TOOK 10 DEEP BREATHS ☐ _____

☐ EXPRESSED GRATITUDE ☐ MEAL PREPPED ☐ PRE-BOLUSED MEALS ☐ _____

☐ SET GOALS FOR TODAY ☐ CARB COUNTED FOOD ☐ SPENT TIME WITH LOVED ONES ☐ _____

EXERCISE: _____

WATER: ☐ ☐ ☐ ☐ ☐ ☐ ☐ ☐ ☐ ☐    TOTAL DAILY INSULIN: _____ UNITS

## THE NIGHT CAP

A PATTERN I RECOGNIZED WAS...

_____

_____

TOMORROW I WANT TO FOCUS MORE ON...

_____

_____

TODAY I CELEBRATE MYSELF BECAUSE...

_____

_____

# MONTH 02 REVIEW + REFLECT

## DIABETES MANAGEMENT SPECIFICS

1. My updated average fasting blood sugar (waking up)? _____

2. My updated current basal insulin:

| TIME OF DAY | MY BASAL |
|---|---|
| 12:00am | |
| | |
| | |
| | |
| | |
| | |
| | |

3. My updated current Insulin: Carb Ratio/s:

| TIME OF DAY | MY ICR |
|---|---|
| 12:00am | |
| | |
| | |
| | |
| | |
| | |
| | |

4. My updated current Insulin Sensitivity Factor/s:

| TIME OF DAY | MY ISF |
|---|---|
| 12:00am | |
| | |
| | |
| | |
| | |
| | |
| | |

5. What actions over the last month have you recognized **best** serve your blood sugars?

_____

_____

6. What actions over the last month have you recognized **least** serve your blood sugars?

_____

_____

# MIND / BODY / SOUL

1.  What changes in your mind, body, or soul are you most proud of so far?

_____

_____

_____

_____

_____

2.  What challenges came up for you this month? Were they in or out of your control? What can you
    learn from them?

_____

_____

_____

_____

# REFINING MY GOALS

Reflect on the three overarching goals you set at the start of the journal. Rewrite (or update if
necessary) your 3 month goals below with new action steps beneath each.

Goal #1: _____

1 SMART Action Step: _____

Goal #2: _____

1 SMART Action Step: _____

Goal #3: _____

1 SMART Action Step: _____

# YOU WERE GIVEN THIS LIFE BECAUSE YOU ARE STRONG ENOUGH TO LIVE IT

# MONTH 03

## WEEKLY CHALLENGE

WEEK 01 _____

_____ ☐ DONE

WEEK 02 _____

_____ ☐ DONE

WEEK 03 _____

_____ ☐ DONE

WEEK 04 _____

_____ ☐ DONE

# MORNING WORK IN

DATE: _____    S / M / T / W / T / F / S

## MINDSET PREP

I AM... _____

ONE THING I'M GRATEFUL FOR IS...

_____

ONE THING I DIDN'T DO YESTERDAY, BUT I WILL DO TODAY...

_____

## DAILY LOG

| TIME | BLOOD SUGAR | OUT OF RANGE (x) | INSULIN | C / F / P | NOTES / FOOD |
|------|-------------|------------------|---------|-----------|--------------|
|      |             |                  |         |           |              |
|      |             |                  |         |           |              |
|      |             |                  |         |           |              |
|      |             |                  |         |           |              |
|      |             |                  |         |           |              |
|      |             |                  |         |           |              |
|      |             |                  |         |           |              |
|      |             |                  |         |           |              |
|      |             |                  |         |           |              |
|      |             |                  |         |           |              |

# EVENING REFLECTION

"Nothing is impossible. The word itself says I AM POSSIBLE."
– Audrey Hepburn

| HOW I FELT | 1 (DISSATISFIED) | 2 | 3 (SO-SO) | 4 | 5 (ON FIRE!) |
|---|---|---|---|---|---|
| MOOD | | | | | |
| ENERGY | | | | | |
| BLOOD SUGAR | | | | | |
| NUTRITION | | | | | |
| MINDSET | | | | | |

## TODAY I...

☐ EXERCISED

☐ MEDITATED

☐ EXPRESSED GRATITUDE

☐ SET GOALS FOR TODAY

☐ CHECKED MY SUGAR EVERY 2 HOURS

☐ WAS MINDFUL WHEN EATING

☐ MEAL PREPPED

☐ CARB COUNTED FOOD

☐ VISUALIZED DAY OF GOOD BLOOD SUGARS

☐ TOOK 10 DEEP BREATHS

☐ PRE-BOLUSED MEALS

☐ SPENT TIME WITH LOVED ONES

☐ TOOK A WALK OUTSIDE

☐ _____

☐ _____

☐ _____

EXERCISE: _____

WATER: ☐ ☐ ☐ ☐ ☐ ☐ ☐ ☐ ☐ ☐     TOTAL DAILY INSULIN: _____ UNITS

## THE NIGHT CAP

A PATTERN I RECOGNIZED WAS...

_____

_____

TOMORROW I WANT TO FOCUS MORE ON...

_____

_____

TODAY I CELEBRATE MYSELF BECAUSE...

_____

_____

# MORNING WORK IN | DATE: _____ S / M / T / W / T / F / S

## MINDSET PREP

I AM... _____

ONE THING I'M GRATEFUL FOR IS...

_____

ONE THING I DIDN'T DO YESTERDAY, BUT I WILL DO TODAY...

_____

## DAILY LOG

| TIME | BLOOD SUGAR | OUT OF RANGE (x) | INSULIN | C / F / P | NOTES / FOOD |
|------|-------------|------------------|---------|-----------|--------------|
|      |             |                  |         |           |              |
|      |             |                  |         |           |              |
|      |             |                  |         |           |              |
|      |             |                  |         |           |              |
|      |             |                  |         |           |              |
|      |             |                  |         |           |              |
|      |             |                  |         |           |              |
|      |             |                  |         |           |              |
|      |             |                  |         |           |              |
|      |             |                  |         |           |              |

# EVENING REFLECTION

"The best way to capture moments is to pay attention. This is how we cultivate mindfulness." – Jon Kabat-Zinn

## HOW I FELT

| | 1 (DISSATISFIED) | 2 | 3 (SO-SO) | 4 | 5 (ON FIRE!) |
|---|---|---|---|---|---|
| MOOD | | | | | |
| ENERGY | | | | | |
| BLOOD SUGAR | | | | | |
| NUTRITION | | | | | |
| MINDSET | | | | | |

## TODAY I...

☐ EXERCISED
☐ MEDITATED
☐ EXPRESSED GRATITUDE
☐ SET GOALS FOR TODAY

☐ CHECKED MY SUGAR EVERY 2 HOURS
☐ WAS MINDFUL WHEN EATING
☐ MEAL PREPPED
☐ CARB COUNTED FOOD

☐ VISUALIZED DAY OF GOOD BLOOD SUGARS
☐ TOOK 10 DEEP BREATHS
☐ PRE-BOLUSED MEALS
☐ SPENT TIME WITH LOVED ONES

☐ TOOK A WALK OUTSIDE
☐ _____
☐ _____
☐ _____

EXERCISE: _____

WATER: ☐ ☐ ☐ ☐ ☐ ☐ ☐ ☐ ☐ ☐          TOTAL DAILY INSULIN: _____ UNITS

## THE NIGHT CAP

A PATTERN I RECOGNIZED WAS...

_____

_____

TOMORROW I WANT TO FOCUS MORE ON...

_____

_____

TODAY I CELEBRATE MYSELF BECAUSE...

_____

_____

# MORNING WORK IN

DATE: _____ S / M / T / W / T / F / S

## MINDSET PREP

I AM... _____

ONE THING I'M GRATEFUL FOR IS...

_____

ONE THING I DIDN'T DO YESTERDAY, BUT I WILL DO TODAY...

_____

## DAILY LOG

| TIME | BLOOD SUGAR | OUT OF RANGE (x) | INSULIN | C / F / P | NOTES / FOOD |
|------|-------------|------------------|---------|-----------|--------------|
|      |             |                  |         |           |              |
|      |             |                  |         |           |              |
|      |             |                  |         |           |              |
|      |             |                  |         |           |              |
|      |             |                  |         |           |              |
|      |             |                  |         |           |              |
|      |             |                  |         |           |              |
|      |             |                  |         |           |              |
|      |             |                  |         |           |              |
|      |             |                  |         |           |              |

# EVENING REFLECTION

"You can't go back and change the beginning, but you can start where you are and change the ending." – C.S. Lewis

| HOW I FELT | 1 (DISSATISFIED) | 2 | 3 (SO-SO) | 4 | 5 (ON FIRE!) |
|---|---|---|---|---|---|
| MOOD | | | | | |
| ENERGY | | | | | |
| BLOOD SUGAR | | | | | |
| NUTRITION | | | | | |
| MINDSET | | | | | |

## TODAY I...

☐ EXERCISED  ☐ CHECKED MY SUGAR EVERY 2 HOURS  ☐ VISUALIZED DAY OF GOOD BLOOD SUGARS  ☐ TOOK A WALK OUTSIDE

☐ MEDITATED  ☐ WAS MINDFUL WHEN EATING  ☐ TOOK 10 DEEP BREATHS  ☐ _____

☐ EXPRESSED GRATITUDE  ☐ MEAL PREPPED  ☐ PRE-BOLUSED MEALS  ☐ _____

☐ SET GOALS FOR TODAY  ☐ CARB COUNTED FOOD  ☐ SPENT TIME WITH LOVED ONES  ☐ _____

EXERCISE: _____

WATER: ☐ ☐ ☐ ☐ ☐ ☐ ☐ ☐ ☐ ☐    TOTAL DAILY INSULIN: _____ UNITS

## THE NIGHT CAP

A PATTERN I RECOGNIZED WAS...

_____

_____

TOMORROW I WANT TO FOCUS MORE ON...

_____

_____

TODAY I CELEBRATE MYSELF BECAUSE...

_____

_____

# MORNING WORK IN | DATE: _____ S / M / T / W / T / F / S

## MINDSET PREP

I AM... _____

ONE THING I'M GRATEFUL FOR IS...

_____

ONE THING I DIDN'T DO YESTERDAY, BUT I WILL DO TODAY...

_____

## DAILY LOG

| TIME | BLOOD SUGAR | OUT OF RANGE (x) | INSULIN | C / F / P | NOTES / FOOD |
|------|-------------|------------------|---------|-----------|--------------|
|      |             |                  |         |           |              |
|      |             |                  |         |           |              |
|      |             |                  |         |           |              |
|      |             |                  |         |           |              |
|      |             |                  |         |           |              |
|      |             |                  |         |           |              |
|      |             |                  |         |           |              |
|      |             |                  |         |           |              |
|      |             |                  |         |           |              |

# EVENING REFLECTION

*A flower does not think to compete with the flower next to it. It just blooms.*

## HOW I FELT

| | 1 (DISSATISFIED) | 2 | 3 (SO-SO) | 4 | 5 (ON FIRE!) |
|---|---|---|---|---|---|
| MOOD | | | | | |
| ENERGY | | | | | |
| BLOOD SUGAR | | | | | |
| NUTRITION | | | | | |
| MINDSET | | | | | |

## TODAY I...

- ☐ EXERCISED
- ☐ CHECKED MY SUGAR EVERY 2 HOURS
- ☐ VISUALIZED DAY OF GOOD BLOOD SUGARS
- ☐ TOOK A WALK OUTSIDE

- ☐ MEDITATED
- ☐ WAS MINDFUL WHEN EATING
- ☐ TOOK 10 DEEP BREATHS
- ☐ _____

- ☐ EXPRESSED GRATITUDE
- ☐ MEAL PREPPED
- ☐ PRE-BOLUSED MEALS
- ☐ _____

- ☐ SET GOALS FOR TODAY
- ☐ CARB COUNTED FOOD
- ☐ SPENT TIME WITH LOVED ONES
- ☐ _____

EXERCISE: _____

WATER: ☐ ☐ ☐ ☐ ☐ ☐ ☐ ☐ ☐ ☐     TOTAL DAILY INSULIN: _____ UNITS

## THE NIGHT CAP

A PATTERN I RECOGNIZED WAS...

_____

_____

TOMORROW I WANT TO FOCUS MORE ON...

_____

_____

TODAY I CELEBRATE MYSELF BECAUSE...

_____

_____

# MORNING WORK IN | DATE: _____ S / M / T / W / T / F / S

## MINDSET PREP

I AM... _____

ONE THING I'M GRATEFUL FOR IS...

_____

ONE THING I DIDN'T DO YESTERDAY, BUT I WILL DO TODAY...

_____

## DAILY LOG

| TIME | BLOOD SUGAR | OUT OF RANGE (x) | INSULIN | C / F / P | NOTES / FOOD |
|------|-------------|------------------|---------|-----------|--------------|
|      |             |                  |         |           |              |
|      |             |                  |         |           |              |
|      |             |                  |         |           |              |
|      |             |                  |         |           |              |
|      |             |                  |         |           |              |
|      |             |                  |         |           |              |
|      |             |                  |         |           |              |
|      |             |                  |         |           |              |
|      |             |                  |         |           |              |
|      |             |                  |         |           |              |

# EVENING REFLECTION

"Whether you think you can or you think you can't, you're right."
– Henry Ford

| HOW I FELT | 1 (DISSATISFIED) | 2 | 3 (SO-SO) | 4 | 5 (ON FIRE!) |
|---|---|---|---|---|---|
| MOOD | | | | | |
| ENERGY | | | | | |
| BLOOD SUGAR | | | | | |
| NUTRITION | | | | | |
| MINDSET | | | | | |

## TODAY I...

- ☐ EXERCISED
- ☐ CHECKED MY SUGAR EVERY 2 HOURS
- ☐ VISUALIZED DAY OF GOOD BLOOD SUGARS
- ☐ TOOK A WALK OUTSIDE

- ☐ MEDITATED
- ☐ WAS MINDFUL WHEN EATING
- ☐ TOOK 10 DEEP BREATHS
- ☐ _____

- ☐ EXPRESSED GRATITUDE
- ☐ MEAL PREPPED
- ☐ PRE-BOLUSED MEALS
- ☐ _____

- ☐ SET GOALS FOR TODAY
- ☐ CARB COUNTED FOOD
- ☐ SPENT TIME WITH LOVED ONES
- ☐ _____

EXERCISE: _____

WATER: ⊔ ⊔ ⊔ ⊔ ⊔ ⊔ ⊔ ⊔ ⊔ ⊔     TOTAL DAILY INSULIN: _____ UNITS

## THE NIGHT CAP

A PATTERN I RECOGNIZED WAS...

_____

_____

TOMORROW I WANT TO FOCUS MORE ON...

_____

_____

TODAY I CELEBRATE MYSELF BECAUSE...

_____

_____

| DATE: _____ S / M / T / W / T / F / S

I AM... _____

ONE THING I'M GRATEFUL FOR IS...

_____

ONE THING I DIDN'T DO YESTERDAY, BUT I WILL DO TODAY...

_____

## DAILY LOG

| TIME | BLOOD SUGAR | OUT OF RANGE (x) | INSULIN | C / F / P | NOTES / FOOD |
|------|-------------|------------------|---------|-----------|--------------|
|      |             |                  |         |           |              |
|      |             |                  |         |           |              |
|      |             |                  |         |           |              |
|      |             |                  |         |           |              |
|      |             |                  |         |           |              |
|      |             |                  |         |           |              |
|      |             |                  |         |           |              |
|      |             |                  |         |           |              |
|      |             |                  |         |           |              |

# EVENING REFLECTION

**JOURNAL PROMPT:**
What can you do less of that will give you more energy and focus?

| HOW I FELT | 1<br>(DISSATISFIED) | 2 | 3<br>(SO-SO) | 4 | 5<br>(ON FIRE!) |
|---|---|---|---|---|---|
| MOOD | | | | | |
| ENERGY | | | | | |
| BLOOD SUGAR | | | | | |
| NUTRITION | | | | | |
| MINDSET | | | | | |

## TODAY I...

- ☐ EXERCISED
- ☐ CHECKED MY SUGAR EVERY 2 HOURS
- ☐ VISUALIZED DAY OF GOOD BLOOD SUGARS
- ☐ TOOK A WALK OUTSIDE

- ☐ MEDITATED
- ☐ WAS MINDFUL WHEN EATING
- ☐ TOOK 10 DEEP BREATHS
- ☐ _____

- ☐ EXPRESSED GRATITUDE
- ☐ MEAL PREPPED
- ☐ PRE-BOLUSED MEALS
- ☐ _____

- ☐ SET GOALS FOR TODAY
- ☐ CARB COUNTED FOOD
- ☐ SPENT TIME WITH LOVED ONES
- ☐ _____

EXERCISE: _____

WATER: ☐ ☐ ☐ ☐ ☐ ☐ ☐ ☐ ☐ ☐     TOTAL DAILY INSULIN: _____ UNITS

## THE NIGHT CAP

A PATTERN I RECOGNIZED WAS...

_____

_____

TOMORROW I WANT TO FOCUS MORE ON...

_____

_____

TODAY I CELEBRATE MYSELF BECAUSE...

_____

_____

# MORNING WORK IN

## MINDSET PREP

I AM... _____

ONE THING I'M GRATEFUL FOR IS...

_____

ONE THING I DIDN'T DO YESTERDAY, BUT I WILL DO TODAY...

_____

## DAILY LOG

| TIME | BLOOD SUGAR | OUT OF RANGE (x) | INSULIN | C / F / P | NOTES / FOOD |
|------|-------------|------------------|---------|-----------|--------------|
|      |             |                  |         |           |              |
|      |             |                  |         |           |              |
|      |             |                  |         |           |              |
|      |             |                  |         |           |              |
|      |             |                  |         |           |              |
|      |             |                  |         |           |              |
|      |             |                  |         |           |              |
|      |             |                  |         |           |              |
|      |             |                  |         |           |              |

# EVENING REFLECTION

"Happiness can be found even in the darkest of times if one only remembers to turn on the light." – Dumbledore

| HOW I FELT | 1 (DISSATISFIED) | 2 | 3 (SO-SO) | 4 | 5 (ON FIRE!) |
|---|---|---|---|---|---|
| MOOD | | | | | |
| ENERGY | | | | | |
| BLOOD SUGAR | | | | | |
| NUTRITION | | | | | |
| MINDSET | | | | | |

## TODAY I...

☐ EXERCISED
☐ MEDITATED
☐ EXPRESSED GRATITUDE
☐ SET GOALS FOR TODAY

☐ CHECKED MY SUGAR EVERY 2 HOURS
☐ WAS MINDFUL WHEN EATING
☐ MEAL PREPPED
☐ CARB COUNTED FOOD

☐ VISUALIZED DAY OF GOOD BLOOD SUGARS
☐ TOOK 10 DEEP BREATHS
☐ PRE-BOLUSED MEALS
☐ SPENT TIME WITH LOVED ONES

☐ TOOK A WALK OUTSIDE
☐ _____
☐ _____
☐ _____

EXERCISE: _____

WATER: ☐ ☐ ☐ ☐ ☐ ☐ ☐ ☐ ☐ ☐     TOTAL DAILY INSULIN: _____ UNITS

## THE NIGHT CAP

A PATTERN I RECOGNIZED WAS...

_____

_____

TOMORROW I WANT TO FOCUS MORE ON...

_____

_____

TODAY I CELEBRATE MYSELF BECAUSE...

_____

_____

# MORNING WORK IN

DATE: _____ S / M / T / W / T / F / S

## MINDSET PREP

I AM... _____

ONE THING I'M GRATEFUL FOR IS...

_____

ONE THING I DIDN'T DO YESTERDAY, BUT I WILL DO TODAY...

_____

## DAILY LOG

| TIME | BLOOD SUGAR | OUT OF RANGE (x) | INSULIN | C / F / P | NOTES / FOOD |
|------|-------------|------------------|---------|-----------|--------------|
|      |             |                  |         |           |              |
|      |             |                  |         |           |              |
|      |             |                  |         |           |              |
|      |             |                  |         |           |              |
|      |             |                  |         |           |              |
|      |             |                  |         |           |              |
|      |             |                  |         |           |              |
|      |             |                  |         |           |              |
|      |             |                  |         |           |              |
|      |             |                  |         |           |              |

# EVENING REFLECTION

"Stop trying to be less of who you are. Let this time in your life cut you open and drain all of the things that are holding you back." – Jennifer Elisabeth

| HOW I FELT | 1 (DISSATISFIED) | 2 | 3 (SO-SO) | 4 | 5 (ON FIRE!) |
|---|---|---|---|---|---|
| MOOD | | | | | |
| ENERGY | | | | | |
| BLOOD SUGAR | | | | | |
| NUTRITION | | | | | |
| MINDSET | | | | | |

## TODAY I...

- ☐ EXERCISED
- ☐ MEDITATED
- ☐ EXPRESSED GRATITUDE
- ☐ SET GOALS FOR TODAY

- ☐ CHECKED MY SUGAR EVERY 2 HOURS
- ☐ WAS MINDFUL WHEN EATING
- ☐ MEAL PREPPED
- ☐ CARB COUNTED FOOD

- ☐ VISUALIZED DAY OF GOOD BLOOD SUGARS
- ☐ TOOK 10 DEEP BREATHS
- ☐ PRE-BOLUSED MEALS
- ☐ SPENT TIME WITH LOVED ONES

- ☐ TOOK A WALK OUTSIDE
- ☐ _____
- ☐ _____
- ☐ _____

EXERCISE: _____

WATER: ☐ ☐ ☐ ☐ ☐ ☐ ☐ ☐ ☐ ☐    TOTAL DAILY INSULIN: _____ UNITS

## THE NIGHT CAP

A PATTERN I RECOGNIZED WAS...

_____

_____

TOMORROW I WANT TO FOCUS MORE ON...

_____

_____

TODAY I CELEBRATE MYSELF BECAUSE...

_____

_____

# MORNING WORK IN

DATE: _____ S / M / T / W / T / F / S

## MINDSET PREP

I AM... _____

ONE THING I'M GRATEFUL FOR IS...

_____

ONE THING I DIDN'T DO YESTERDAY, BUT I WILL DO TODAY...

_____

## DAILY LOG

| TIME | BLOOD SUGAR | OUT OF RANGE (x) | INSULIN | C / F / P | NOTES / FOOD |
|------|-------------|------------------|---------|-----------|--------------|
|      |             |                  |         |           |              |
|      |             |                  |         |           |              |
|      |             |                  |         |           |              |
|      |             |                  |         |           |              |
|      |             |                  |         |           |              |
|      |             |                  |         |           |              |
|      |             |                  |         |           |              |
|      |             |                  |         |           |              |
|      |             |                  |         |           |              |
|      |             |                  |         |           |              |

# EVENING REFLECTION

"Don't believe everything you think. Thoughts are just that – thoughts." – Allan Lokos

| HOW I FELT | 1 (DISSATISFIED) | 2 | 3 (SO-SO) | 4 | 5 (ON FIRE!) |
|---|---|---|---|---|---|
| MOOD | | | | | |
| ENERGY | | | | | |
| BLOOD SUGAR | | | | | |
| NUTRITION | | | | | |
| MINDSET | | | | | |

## TODAY I...

☐ EXERCISED

☐ MEDITATED

☐ EXPRESSED GRATITUDE

☐ SET GOALS FOR TODAY

☐ CHECKED MY SUGAR EVERY 2 HOURS

☐ WAS MINDFUL WHEN EATING

☐ MEAL PREPPED

☐ CARB COUNTED FOOD

☐ VISUALIZED DAY OF GOOD BLOOD SUGARS

☐ TOOK 10 DEEP BREATHS

☐ PRE-BOLUSED MEALS

☐ SPENT TIME WITH LOVED ONES

☐ TOOK A WALK OUTSIDE

☐ _____

☐ _____

☐ _____

EXERCISE: _____

WATER: ☐ ☐ ☐ ☐ ☐ ☐ ☐ ☐ ☐ ☐        TOTAL DAILY INSULIN: _____ UNITS

## THE NIGHT CAP

A PATTERN I RECOGNIZED WAS...

_____

_____

TOMORROW I WANT TO FOCUS MORE ON...

_____

_____

TODAY I CELEBRATE MYSELF BECAUSE...

_____

_____

# MORNING WORK IN

## MINDSET PREP

I AM... _____

ONE THING I'M GRATEFUL FOR IS...

_____

ONE THING I DIDN'T DO YESTERDAY, BUT I WILL DO TODAY...

_____

## DAILY LOG

| TIME | BLOOD SUGAR | OUT OF RANGE (x) | INSULIN | C / F / P | NOTES / FOOD |
|------|-------------|------------------|---------|-----------|--------------|
|      |             |                  |         |           |              |
|      |             |                  |         |           |              |
|      |             |                  |         |           |              |
|      |             |                  |         |           |              |
|      |             |                  |         |           |              |
|      |             |                  |         |           |              |
|      |             |                  |         |           |              |
|      |             |                  |         |           |              |
|      |             |                  |         |           |              |

# EVENING REFLECTION | *Keep your body clean, it's the house to your soul.*

## HOW I FELT

| | 1 (DISSATISFIED) | 2 | 3 (SO-SO) | 4 | 5 (ON FIRE!) |
|---|---|---|---|---|---|
| MOOD | | | | | |
| ENERGY | | | | | |
| BLOOD SUGAR | | | | | |
| NUTRITION | | | | | |
| MINDSET | | | | | |

## TODAY I...

☐ EXERCISED    ☐ CHECKED MY SUGAR EVERY 2 HOURS    ☐ VISUALIZED DAY OF GOOD BLOOD SUGARS    ☐ TOOK A WALK OUTSIDE

☐ MEDITATED    ☐ WAS MINDFUL WHEN EATING    ☐ TOOK 10 DEEP BREATHS    ☐ _____

☐ EXPRESSED GRATITUDE    ☐ MEAL PREPPED    ☐ PRE-BOLUSED MEALS    ☐ _____

☐ SET GOALS FOR TODAY    ☐ CARB COUNTED FOOD    ☐ SPENT TIME WITH LOVED ONES    ☐ _____

EXERCISE: _____

WATER: ☐ ☐ ☐ ☐ ☐ ☐ ☐ ☐ ☐ ☐    TOTAL DAILY INSULIN: _____ UNITS

## THE NIGHT CAP

A PATTERN I RECOGNIZED WAS...

_____

_____

TOMORROW I WANT TO FOCUS MORE ON...

_____

_____

TODAY I CELEBRATE MYSELF BECAUSE...

_____

_____

# MORNING WORK IN

DATE: _____     S / M / T / W / T / F / S

## MINDSET PREP

I AM... _____

ONE THING I'M GRATEFUL FOR IS...

_____

ONE THING I DIDN'T DO YESTERDAY, BUT I WILL DO TODAY...

_____

## DAILY LOG

| TIME | BLOOD SUGAR | OUT OF RANGE (x) | INSULIN | C / F / P | NOTES / FOOD |
|------|-------------|------------------|---------|-----------|--------------|
|      |             |                  |         |           |              |
|      |             |                  |         |           |              |
|      |             |                  |         |           |              |
|      |             |                  |         |           |              |
|      |             |                  |         |           |              |
|      |             |                  |         |           |              |
|      |             |                  |         |           |              |
|      |             |                  |         |           |              |
|      |             |                  |         |           |              |

# EVENING REFLECTION

"We chase what we want but sometimes we need to chase what we need." – Jon Taffer

| HOW I FELT | 1 (DISSATISFIED) | 2 | 3 (SO-SO) | 4 | 5 (ON FIRE!) |
|---|---|---|---|---|---|
| MOOD | | | | | |
| ENERGY | | | | | |
| BLOOD SUGAR | | | | | |
| NUTRITION | | | | | |
| MINDSET | | | | | |

## TODAY I...

- ☐ EXERCISED
- ☐ MEDITATED
- ☐ EXPRESSED GRATITUDE
- ☐ SET GOALS FOR TODAY

- ☐ CHECKED MY SUGAR EVERY 2 HOURS
- ☐ WAS MINDFUL WHEN EATING
- ☐ MEAL PREPPED
- ☐ CARB COUNTED FOOD

- ☐ VISUALIZED DAY OF GOOD BLOOD SUGARS
- ☐ TOOK 10 DEEP BREATHS
- ☐ PRE-BOLUSED MEALS
- ☐ SPENT TIME WITH LOVED ONES

- ☐ TOOK A WALK OUTSIDE
- ☐ _____
- ☐ _____
- ☐ _____

EXERCISE: _____

WATER: ▯ ▯ ▯ ▯ ▯ ▯ ▯ ▯ ▯ ▯    TOTAL DAILY INSULIN: _____ UNITS

## THE NIGHT CAP

A PATTERN I RECOGNIZED WAS...

_____

_____

TOMORROW I WANT TO FOCUS MORE ON...

_____

_____

TODAY I CELEBRATE MYSELF BECAUSE...

_____

_____

# MORNING WORK IN

DATE: _____     S / M / T / W / T / F / S

## MINDSET PREP

I AM... _____

ONE THING I'M GRATEFUL FOR IS...

_____

ONE THING I DIDN'T DO YESTERDAY, BUT I WILL DO TODAY...

_____

## DAILY LOG

| TIME | BLOOD SUGAR | OUT OF RANGE (x) | INSULIN | C / F / P | NOTES / FOOD |
|------|-------------|------------------|---------|-----------|--------------|
|      |             |                  |         |           |              |
|      |             |                  |         |           |              |
|      |             |                  |         |           |              |
|      |             |                  |         |           |              |
|      |             |                  |         |           |              |
|      |             |                  |         |           |              |
|      |             |                  |         |           |              |
|      |             |                  |         |           |              |
|      |             |                  |         |           |              |
|      |             |                  |         |           |              |

# EVENING REFLECTION

**JOURNAL PROMPT:**
What is weighing heavy on your heart this week? What do you need to do to release it?

| HOW I FELT | 1 (DISSATISFIED) | 2 | 3 (SO-SO) | 4 | 5 (ON FIRE!) |
|---|---|---|---|---|---|
| MOOD | | | | | |
| ENERGY | | | | | |
| BLOOD SUGAR | | | | | |
| NUTRITION | | | | | |
| MINDSET | | | | | |

## TODAY I...

- ☐ EXERCISED
- ☐ MEDITATED
- ☐ EXPRESSED GRATITUDE
- ☐ SET GOALS FOR TODAY

- ☐ CHECKED MY SUGAR EVERY 2 HOURS
- ☐ WAS MINDFUL WHEN EATING
- ☐ MEAL PREPPED
- ☐ CARB COUNTED FOOD

- ☐ VISUALIZED DAY OF GOOD BLOOD SUGARS
- ☐ TOOK 10 DEEP BREATHS
- ☐ PRE-BOLUSED MEALS
- ☐ SPENT TIME WITH LOVED ONES

- ☐ TOOK A WALK OUTSIDE
- ☐ _____
- ☐ _____
- ☐ _____

EXERCISE: _____

WATER: ☐ ☐ ☐ ☐ ☐ ☐ ☐ ☐ ☐ ☐        TOTAL DAILY INSULIN: _____ UNITS

## THE NIGHT CAP

A PATTERN I RECOGNIZED WAS...

_____

_____

TOMORROW I WANT TO FOCUS MORE ON...

_____

_____

TODAY I CELEBRATE MYSELF BECAUSE...

_____

_____

# MORNING WORK IN | DATE: _____ S / M / T / W / T / F / S

## MINDSET PREP

I AM... _____

ONE THING I'M GRATEFUL FOR IS...

_____

ONE THING I DIDN'T DO YESTERDAY, BUT I WILL DO TODAY...

_____

## DAILY LOG

| TIME | BLOOD SUGAR | OUT OF RANGE (x) | INSULIN | C / F / P | NOTES / FOOD |
|------|-------------|------------------|---------|-----------|--------------|
|      |             |                  |         |           |              |
|      |             |                  |         |           |              |
|      |             |                  |         |           |              |
|      |             |                  |         |           |              |
|      |             |                  |         |           |              |
|      |             |                  |         |           |              |
|      |             |                  |         |           |              |
|      |             |                  |         |           |              |
|      |             |                  |         |           |              |

# EVENING REFLECTION

"Gratitude unlocks the fullness of life. It turns what we have into enough, and more." – Melody Beattie

## HOW I FELT

| | 1 (DISSATISFIED) | 2 | 3 (SO-SO) | 4 | 5 (ON FIRE!) |
|---|---|---|---|---|---|
| MOOD | | | | | |
| ENERGY | | | | | |
| BLOOD SUGAR | | | | | |
| NUTRITION | | | | | |
| MINDSET | | | | | |

## TODAY I...

- [ ] EXERCISED
- [ ] MEDITATED
- [ ] EXPRESSED GRATITUDE
- [ ] SET GOALS FOR TODAY

- [ ] CHECKED MY SUGAR EVERY 2 HOURS
- [ ] WAS MINDFUL WHEN EATING
- [ ] MEAL PREPPED
- [ ] CARB COUNTED FOOD

- [ ] VISUALIZED DAY OF GOOD BLOOD SUGARS
- [ ] TOOK 10 DEEP BREATHS
- [ ] PRE-BOLUSED MEALS
- [ ] SPENT TIME WITH LOVED ONES

- [ ] TOOK A WALK OUTSIDE
- [ ] _____
- [ ] _____
- [ ] _____

EXERCISE: _____

WATER: ⬜ ⬜ ⬜ ⬜ ⬜ ⬜ ⬜ ⬜ ⬜ ⬜      TOTAL DAILY INSULIN: _____ UNITS

## THE NIGHT CAP

A PATTERN I RECOGNIZED WAS...

_____

_____

TOMORROW I WANT TO FOCUS MORE ON...

_____

_____

TODAY I CELEBRATE MYSELF BECAUSE...

_____

_____

# MORNING WORK IN

## MINDSET PREP

I AM... _____

ONE THING I'M GRATEFUL FOR IS...

_____

ONE THING I DIDN'T DO YESTERDAY, BUT I WILL DO TODAY...

_____

## DAILY LOG

| TIME | BLOOD SUGAR | OUT OF RANGE (x) | INSULIN | C / F / P | NOTES / FOOD |
|------|-------------|------------------|---------|-----------|--------------|
|      |             |                  |         |           |              |
|      |             |                  |         |           |              |
|      |             |                  |         |           |              |
|      |             |                  |         |           |              |
|      |             |                  |         |           |              |
|      |             |                  |         |           |              |
|      |             |                  |         |           |              |
|      |             |                  |         |           |              |
|      |             |                  |         |           |              |
|      |             |                  |         |           |              |

# EVENING REFLECTION | "You cannot control the results, only your actions." – Allan Lokos

| HOW I FELT | 1<br>(DISSATISFIED) | 2 | 3<br>(SO-SO) | 4 | 5<br>(ON FIRE!) |
|---|---|---|---|---|---|
| MOOD | | | | | |
| ENERGY | | | | | |
| BLOOD SUGAR | | | | | |
| NUTRITION | | | | | |
| MINDSET | | | | | |

## TODAY I...

- ☐ EXERCISED
- ☐ MEDITATED
- ☐ EXPRESSED GRATITUDE
- ☐ SET GOALS FOR TODAY

- ☐ CHECKED MY SUGAR EVERY 2 HOURS
- ☐ WAS MINDFUL WHEN EATING
- ☐ MEAL PREPPED
- ☐ CARB COUNTED FOOD

- ☐ VISUALIZED DAY OF GOOD BLOOD SUGARS
- ☐ TOOK 10 DEEP BREATHS
- ☐ PRE-BOLUSED MEALS
- ☐ SPENT TIME WITH LOVED ONES

- ☐ TOOK A WALK OUTSIDE
- ☐ _____
- ☐ _____
- ☐ _____

EXERCISE: _____

WATER: ⊔ ⊔ ⊔ ⊔ ⊔ ⊔ ⊔ ⊔ ⊔ ⊔     TOTAL DAILY INSULIN: _____ UNITS

## THE NIGHT CAP

A PATTERN I RECOGNIZED WAS...

_____

_____

TOMORROW I WANT TO FOCUS MORE ON...

_____

_____

TODAY I CELEBRATE MYSELF BECAUSE...

_____

_____

# MORNING WORK IN | DATE: _____ S / M / T / W / T / F / S

## MINDSET PREP

I AM... _____

ONE THING I'M GRATEFUL FOR IS...

_____

ONE THING I DIDN'T DO YESTERDAY, BUT I WILL DO TODAY...

_____

## DAILY LOG

| TIME | BLOOD SUGAR | OUT OF RANGE (x) | INSULIN | C / F / P | NOTES / FOOD |
|------|-------------|------------------|---------|-----------|--------------|
|      |             |                  |         |           |              |
|      |             |                  |         |           |              |
|      |             |                  |         |           |              |
|      |             |                  |         |           |              |
|      |             |                  |         |           |              |
|      |             |                  |         |           |              |
|      |             |                  |         |           |              |
|      |             |                  |         |           |              |
|      |             |                  |         |           |              |
|      |             |                  |         |           |              |

# EVENING REFLECTION

"The key is to go from '*I can't do something*' to '*why can't I.*'"
– LNB

| HOW I FELT | 1 (DISSATISFIED) | 2 | 3 (SO-SO) | 4 | 5 (ON FIRE!) |
|---|---|---|---|---|---|
| MOOD | | | | | |
| ENERGY | | | | | |
| BLOOD SUGAR | | | | | |
| NUTRITION | | | | | |
| MINDSET | | | | | |

## TODAY I...

- ☐ EXERCISED
- ☐ MEDITATED
- ☐ EXPRESSED GRATITUDE
- ☐ SET GOALS FOR TODAY

- ☐ CHECKED MY SUGAR EVERY 2 HOURS
- ☐ WAS MINDFUL WHEN EATING
- ☐ MEAL PREPPED
- ☐ CARB COUNTED FOOD

- ☐ VISUALIZED DAY OF GOOD BLOOD SUGARS
- ☐ TOOK 10 DEEP BREATHS
- ☐ PRE-BOLUSED MEALS
- ☐ SPENT TIME WITH LOVED ONES

- ☐ TOOK A WALK OUTSIDE
- ☐ _____
- ☐ _____
- ☐ _____

EXERCISE: _____

WATER: ⊔ ⊔ ⊔ ⊔ ⊔ ⊔ ⊔ ⊔ ⊔ ⊔          TOTAL DAILY INSULIN: _____ UNITS

## THE NIGHT CAP

A PATTERN I RECOGNIZED WAS...

_____

_____

TOMORROW I WANT TO FOCUS MORE ON...

_____

_____

TODAY I CELEBRATE MYSELF BECAUSE...

_____

_____

# MORNING WORK IN

DATE: _____ S / M / T / W / T / F / S

## MINDSET PREP

I AM... _____

ONE THING I'M GRATEFUL FOR IS...

_____

ONE THING I DIDN'T DO YESTERDAY, BUT I WILL DO TODAY...

_____

## DAILY LOG

| TIME | BLOOD SUGAR | OUT OF RANGE (x) | INSULIN | C / F / P | NOTES / FOOD |
|------|-------------|------------------|---------|-----------|--------------|
|      |             |                  |         |           |              |
|      |             |                  |         |           |              |
|      |             |                  |         |           |              |
|      |             |                  |         |           |              |
|      |             |                  |         |           |              |
|      |             |                  |         |           |              |
|      |             |                  |         |           |              |
|      |             |                  |         |           |              |
|      |             |                  |         |           |              |

# EVENING REFLECTION | "Nothing will work unless you do." – Maya Angelou

| HOW I FELT | 1 (DISSATISFIED) | 2 | 3 (SO-SO) | 4 | 5 (ON FIRE!) |
|---|---|---|---|---|---|
| MOOD | | | | | |
| ENERGY | | | | | |
| BLOOD SUGAR | | | | | |
| NUTRITION | | | | | |
| MINDSET | | | | | |

## TODAY I...

☐ EXERCISED    ☐ CHECKED MY SUGAR EVERY 2 HOURS    ☐ VISUALIZED DAY OF GOOD BLOOD SUGARS    ☐ TOOK A WALK OUTSIDE

☐ MEDITATED    ☐ WAS MINDFUL WHEN EATING    ☐ TOOK 10 DEEP BREATHS    ☐ _____

☐ EXPRESSED GRATITUDE    ☐ MEAL PREPPED    ☐ PRE-BOLUSED MEALS    ☐ _____

☐ SET GOALS FOR TODAY    ☐ CARB COUNTED FOOD    ☐ SPENT TIME WITH LOVED ONES    ☐ _____

EXERCISE: _____

WATER: ▯ ▯ ▯ ▯ ▯ ▯ ▯ ▯ ▯ ▯    TOTAL DAILY INSULIN: _____ UNITS

## THE NIGHT CAP

A PATTERN I RECOGNIZED WAS...

_____

_____

TOMORROW I WANT TO FOCUS MORE ON...

_____

_____

TODAY I CELEBRATE MYSELF BECAUSE...

_____

_____

# MORNING WORK IN

## MINDSET PREP

I AM... _____

ONE THING I'M GRATEFUL FOR IS...

_____

ONE THING I DIDN'T DO YESTERDAY, BUT I WILL DO TODAY...

_____

## DAILY LOG

| TIME | BLOOD SUGAR | OUT OF RANGE (x) | INSULIN | C / F / P | NOTES / FOOD |
|------|-------------|------------------|---------|-----------|--------------|
|      |             |                  |         |           |              |
|      |             |                  |         |           |              |
|      |             |                  |         |           |              |
|      |             |                  |         |           |              |
|      |             |                  |         |           |              |
|      |             |                  |         |           |              |
|      |             |                  |         |           |              |
|      |             |                  |         |           |              |
|      |             |                  |         |           |              |

# EVENING REFLECTION

"Meditation is not evasion; it is a serene encounter with reality."
– Thích Nhất Hạnh

## HOW I FELT

| | 1 (DISSATISFIED) | 2 | 3 (SO-SO) | 4 | 5 (ON FIRE!) |
|---|---|---|---|---|---|
| MOOD | | | | | |
| ENERGY | | | | | |
| BLOOD SUGAR | | | | | |
| NUTRITION | | | | | |
| MINDSET | | | | | |

## TODAY I...

- [ ] EXERCISED
- [ ] MEDITATED
- [ ] EXPRESSED GRATITUDE
- [ ] SET GOALS FOR TODAY

- [ ] CHECKED MY SUGAR EVERY 2 HOURS
- [ ] WAS MINDFUL WHEN EATING
- [ ] MEAL PREPPED
- [ ] CARB COUNTED FOOD

- [ ] VISUALIZED DAY OF GOOD BLOOD SUGARS
- [ ] TOOK 10 DEEP BREATHS
- [ ] PRE-BOLUSED MEALS
- [ ] SPENT TIME WITH LOVED ONES

- [ ] TOOK A WALK OUTSIDE
- [ ] _____
- [ ] _____
- [ ] _____

EXERCISE: _____

WATER: ⬜ ⬜ ⬜ ⬜ ⬜ ⬜ ⬜ ⬜ ⬜ ⬜          TOTAL DAILY INSULIN: _____ UNITS

## THE NIGHT CAP

A PATTERN I RECOGNIZED WAS...

_____

_____

TOMORROW I WANT TO FOCUS MORE ON...

_____

_____

TODAY I CELEBRATE MYSELF BECAUSE...

_____

_____

# MORNING WORK IN

DATE: _____ S / M / T / W / T / F / S

## MINDSET PREP

I AM... _____

ONE THING I'M GRATEFUL FOR IS...

_____

ONE THING I DIDN'T DO YESTERDAY, BUT I WILL DO TODAY...

_____

## DAILY LOG

| TIME | BLOOD SUGAR | OUT OF RANGE (x) | INSULIN | C / F / P | NOTES / FOOD |
|------|-------------|------------------|---------|-----------|--------------|
|      |             |                  |         |           |              |
|      |             |                  |         |           |              |
|      |             |                  |         |           |              |
|      |             |                  |         |           |              |
|      |             |                  |         |           |              |
|      |             |                  |         |           |              |
|      |             |                  |         |           |              |
|      |             |                  |         |           |              |
|      |             |                  |         |           |              |
|      |             |                  |         |           |              |

# EVENING REFLECTION

"Our lives will remain the same unless we shift in the mind, shift in the action, and understand that we need to meet our potential halfway." – LNB

| HOW I FELT | 1 (DISSATISFIED) | 2 | 3 (SO-SO) | 4 | 5 (ON FIRE!) |
|---|---|---|---|---|---|
| MOOD | | | | | |
| ENERGY | | | | | |
| BLOOD SUGAR | | | | | |
| NUTRITION | | | | | |
| MINDSET | | | | | |

## TODAY I...

- [ ] EXERCISED
- [ ] MEDITATED
- [ ] EXPRESSED GRATITUDE
- [ ] SET GOALS FOR TODAY

- [ ] CHECKED MY SUGAR EVERY 2 HOURS
- [ ] WAS MINDFUL WHEN EATING
- [ ] MEAL PREPPED
- [ ] CARB COUNTED FOOD

- [ ] VISUALIZED DAY OF GOOD BLOOD SUGARS
- [ ] TOOK 10 DEEP BREATHS
- [ ] PRE-BOLUSED MEALS
- [ ] SPENT TIME WITH LOVED ONES

- [ ] TOOK A WALK OUTSIDE
- [ ] _____
- [ ] _____
- [ ] _____

EXERCISE: _____

WATER: ⛛ ⛛ ⛛ ⛛ ⛛ ⛛ ⛛ ⛛ ⛛ ⛛     TOTAL DAILY INSULIN: _____ UNITS

## THE NIGHT CAP

A PATTERN I RECOGNIZED WAS...

_____

_____

TOMORROW I WANT TO FOCUS MORE ON...

_____

_____

TODAY I CELEBRATE MYSELF BECAUSE...

_____

_____

# MORNING WORK IN

DATE: _____ S / M / T / W / T / F / S

I AM... _____

ONE THING I'M GRATEFUL FOR IS...

_____

ONE THING I DIDN'T DO YESTERDAY, BUT I WILL DO TODAY...

_____

## DAILY LOG

| TIME | BLOOD SUGAR | OUT OF RANGE (x) | INSULIN | C / F / P | NOTES / FOOD |
|------|-------------|------------------|---------|-----------|--------------|
|      |             |                  |         |           |              |
|      |             |                  |         |           |              |
|      |             |                  |         |           |              |
|      |             |                  |         |           |              |
|      |             |                  |         |           |              |
|      |             |                  |         |           |              |
|      |             |                  |         |           |              |
|      |             |                  |         |           |              |
|      |             |                  |         |           |              |

# EVENING REFLECTION | "That's life: starting over, one breath at a time." – Sharon Salzberg

| HOW I FELT | 1 (DISSATISFIED) | 2 | 3 (SO-SO) | 4 | 5 (ON FIRE!) |
|---|---|---|---|---|---|
| MOOD | | | | | |
| ENERGY | | | | | |
| BLOOD SUGAR | | | | | |
| NUTRITION | | | | | |
| MINDSET | | | | | |

## TODAY I...

☐ EXERCISED    ☐ CHECKED MY SUGAR EVERY 2 HOURS    ☐ VISUALIZED DAY OF GOOD BLOOD SUGARS    ☐ TOOK A WALK OUTSIDE

☐ MEDITATED    ☐ WAS MINDFUL WHEN EATING    ☐ TOOK 10 DEEP BREATHS    ☐ _____

☐ EXPRESSED GRATITUDE    ☐ MEAL PREPPED    ☐ PRE-BOLUSED MEALS    ☐ _____

☐ SET GOALS FOR TODAY    ☐ CARB COUNTED FOOD    ☐ SPENT TIME WITH LOVED ONES    ☐ _____

EXERCISE: _____

WATER: ⊔ ⊔ ⊔ ⊔ ⊔ ⊔ ⊔ ⊔ ⊔ ⊔    TOTAL DAILY INSULIN: _____ UNITS

## THE NIGHT CAP

A PATTERN I RECOGNIZED WAS...

_____

_____

TOMORROW I WANT TO FOCUS MORE ON...

_____

_____

TODAY I CELEBRATE MYSELF BECAUSE...

_____

_____

# MORNING WORK IN | DATE: _____  S / M / T / W / T / F / S

## MINDSET PREP

I AM... _____

ONE THING I'M GRATEFUL FOR IS...

_____

ONE THING I DIDN'T DO YESTERDAY, BUT I WILL DO TODAY...

_____

## DAILY LOG

| TIME | BLOOD SUGAR | OUT OF RANGE (x) | INSULIN | C / F / P | NOTES / FOOD |
|------|-------------|------------------|---------|-----------|--------------|
|      |             |                  |         |           |              |
|      |             |                  |         |           |              |
|      |             |                  |         |           |              |
|      |             |                  |         |           |              |
|      |             |                  |         |           |              |
|      |             |                  |         |           |              |
|      |             |                  |         |           |              |
|      |             |                  |         |           |              |
|      |             |                  |         |           |              |
|      |             |                  |         |           |              |

# EVENING REFLECTION

**JOURNAL PROMPT:**
What would today look like if you were living as your highest self?

| HOW I FELT | 1 (DISSATISFIED) | 2 | 3 (SO-SO) | 4 | 5 (ON FIRE!) |
|---|---|---|---|---|---|
| MOOD | | | | | |
| ENERGY | | | | | |
| BLOOD SUGAR | | | | | |
| NUTRITION | | | | | |
| MINDSET | | | | | |

## TODAY I...

☐ EXERCISED

☐ MEDITATED

☐ EXPRESSED GRATITUDE

☐ SET GOALS FOR TODAY

☐ CHECKED MY SUGAR EVERY 2 HOURS

☐ WAS MINDFUL WHEN EATING

☐ MEAL PREPPED

☐ CARB COUNTED FOOD

☐ VISUALIZED DAY OF GOOD BLOOD SUGARS

☐ TOOK 10 DEEP BREATHS

☐ PRE-BOLUSED MEALS

☐ SPENT TIME WITH LOVED ONES

☐ TOOK A WALK OUTSIDE

☐ _____

☐ _____

☐ _____

EXERCISE: _____

WATER: ▽ ▽ ▽ ▽ ▽ ▽ ▽ ▽ ▽ ▽     TOTAL DAILY INSULIN: _____ UNITS

## THE NIGHT CAP

A PATTERN I RECOGNIZED WAS...

_____

_____

TOMORROW I WANT TO FOCUS MORE ON...

_____

_____

TODAY I CELEBRATE MYSELF BECAUSE...

_____

_____

# MORNING WORK IN

DATE: _____   S / M / T / W / T / F / S

I AM... _____

ONE THING I'M GRATEFUL FOR IS...

_____

ONE THING I DIDN'T DO YESTERDAY, BUT I WILL DO TODAY...

_____

## DAILY LOG

| TIME | BLOOD SUGAR | OUT OF RANGE (x) | INSULIN | C / F / P | NOTES / FOOD |
|------|-------------|------------------|---------|-----------|--------------|
|      |             |                  |         |           |              |
|      |             |                  |         |           |              |
|      |             |                  |         |           |              |
|      |             |                  |         |           |              |
|      |             |                  |         |           |              |
|      |             |                  |         |           |              |
|      |             |                  |         |           |              |
|      |             |                  |         |           |              |
|      |             |                  |         |           |              |
|      |             |                  |         |           |              |

# EVENING REFLECTION

"In your own life it's important to know how spectacular you are."
– Steve Maraboli

| HOW I FELT | 1 (DISSATISFIED) | 2 | 3 (SO-SO) | 4 | 5 (ON FIRE!) |
|---|---|---|---|---|---|
| MOOD | | | | | |
| ENERGY | | | | | |
| BLOOD SUGAR | | | | | |
| NUTRITION | | | | | |
| MINDSET | | | | | |

## TODAY I...

☐ EXERCISED

☐ MEDITATED

☐ EXPRESSED GRATITUDE

☐ SET GOALS FOR TODAY

☐ CHECKED MY SUGAR EVERY 2 HOURS

☐ WAS MINDFUL WHEN EATING

☐ MEAL PREPPED

☐ CARB COUNTED FOOD

☐ VISUALIZED DAY OF GOOD BLOOD SUGARS

☐ TOOK 10 DEEP BREATHS

☐ PRE-BOLUSED MEALS

☐ SPENT TIME WITH LOVED ONES

☐ TOOK A WALK OUTSIDE

☐ _____

☐ _____

☐ _____

EXERCISE: _____

WATER: ▽ ▽ ▽ ▽ ▽ ▽ ▽ ▽ ▽ ▽     TOTAL DAILY INSULIN: _____ UNITS

## THE NIGHT CAP

A PATTERN I RECOGNIZED WAS...

_____

_____

TOMORROW I WANT TO FOCUS MORE ON...

_____

_____

TODAY I CELEBRATE MYSELF BECAUSE...

_____

_____

# MORNING WORK IN | DATE: _____ / _____ S / M / T / W / T / F / S

## MINDSET PREP

I AM... _____

ONE THING I'M GRATEFUL FOR IS...

_____

ONE THING I DIDN'T DO YESTERDAY, BUT I WILL DO TODAY...

_____

## DAILY LOG

| TIME | BLOOD SUGAR | OUT OF RANGE (x) | INSULIN | C / F / P | NOTES / FOOD |
|------|-------------|------------------|---------|-----------|--------------|
|      |             |                  |         |           |              |
|      |             |                  |         |           |              |
|      |             |                  |         |           |              |
|      |             |                  |         |           |              |
|      |             |                  |         |           |              |
|      |             |                  |         |           |              |
|      |             |                  |         |           |              |
|      |             |                  |         |           |              |
|      |             |                  |         |           |              |

# EVENING REFLECTION

"Your actions are your only true belongings." – Allan Lokos

| HOW I FELT | 1 (DISSATISFIED) | 2 | 3 (SO-SO) | 4 | 5 (ON FIRE!) |
|---|---|---|---|---|---|
| MOOD | | | | | |
| ENERGY | | | | | |
| BLOOD SUGAR | | | | | |
| NUTRITION | | | | | |
| MINDSET | | | | | |

## TODAY I...

- [ ] EXERCISED
- [ ] MEDITATED
- [ ] EXPRESSED GRATITUDE
- [ ] SET GOALS FOR TODAY

- [ ] CHECKED MY SUGAR EVERY 2 HOURS
- [ ] WAS MINDFUL WHEN EATING
- [ ] MEAL PREPPED
- [ ] CARB COUNTED FOOD

- [ ] VISUALIZED DAY OF GOOD BLOOD SUGARS
- [ ] TOOK 10 DEEP BREATHS
- [ ] PRE-BOLUSED MEALS
- [ ] SPENT TIME WITH LOVED ONES

- [ ] TOOK A WALK OUTSIDE
- [ ] _____
- [ ] _____
- [ ] _____

EXERCISE: _____

WATER: ⊔ ⊔ ⊔ ⊔ ⊔ ⊔ ⊔ ⊔ ⊔ ⊔     TOTAL DAILY INSULIN: _____ UNITS

## THE NIGHT CAP

A PATTERN I RECOGNIZED WAS...

_____

_____

TOMORROW I WANT TO FOCUS MORE ON...

_____

_____

TODAY I CELEBRATE MYSELF BECAUSE...

_____

_____

# MORNING WORK IN | DATE: _____ S / M / T / W / T / F / S

I AM... _____

ONE THING I'M GRATEFUL FOR IS...

_____

ONE THING I DIDN'T DO YESTERDAY, BUT I WILL DO TODAY...

_____

## DAILY LOG

| TIME | BLOOD SUGAR | OUT OF RANGE (x) | INSULIN | C / F / P | NOTES / FOOD |
|------|-------------|------------------|---------|-----------|--------------|
|      |             |                  |         |           |              |
|      |             |                  |         |           |              |
|      |             |                  |         |           |              |
|      |             |                  |         |           |              |
|      |             |                  |         |           |              |
|      |             |                  |         |           |              |
|      |             |                  |         |           |              |
|      |             |                  |         |           |              |
|      |             |                  |         |           |              |

# EVENING REFLECTION

"When we get too caught up in the busyness of the world, we lose connection with one another – and ourselves."
– Jack Kornfield

| HOW I FELT | 1 (DISSATISFIED) | 2 | 3 (SO-SO) | 4 | 5 (ON FIRE!) |
|---|---|---|---|---|---|
| MOOD | | | | | |
| ENERGY | | | | | |
| BLOOD SUGAR | | | | | |
| NUTRITION | | | | | |
| MINDSET | | | | | |

## TODAY I...

☐ EXERCISED

☐ MEDITATED

☐ EXPRESSED GRATITUDE

☐ SET GOALS FOR TODAY

☐ CHECKED MY SUGAR EVERY 2 HOURS

☐ WAS MINDFUL WHEN EATING

☐ MEAL PREPPED

☐ CARB COUNTED FOOD

☐ VISUALIZED DAY OF GOOD BLOOD SUGARS

☐ TOOK 10 DEEP BREATHS

☐ PRE-BOLUSED MEALS

☐ SPENT TIME WITH LOVED ONES

☐ TOOK A WALK OUTSIDE

☐ _____

☐ _____

☐ _____

EXERCISE: _____

WATER: ▽ ▽ ▽ ▽ ▽ ▽ ▽ ▽ ▽ ▽     TOTAL DAILY INSULIN: _____ UNITS

## THE NIGHT CAP

A PATTERN I RECOGNIZED WAS...

_____

_____

TOMORROW I WANT TO FOCUS MORE ON...

_____

_____

TODAY I CELEBRATE MYSELF BECAUSE...

_____

_____

# MORNING WORK IN | DATE: _____ S / M / T / W / T / F / S

## MINDSET PREP

I AM... _____

ONE THING I'M GRATEFUL FOR IS...

_____

ONE THING I DIDN'T DO YESTERDAY, BUT I WILL DO TODAY...

_____

## DAILY LOG

| TIME | BLOOD SUGAR | OUT OF RANGE (x) | INSULIN | C / F / P | NOTES / FOOD |
|------|-------------|------------------|---------|-----------|--------------|
|      |             |                  |         |           |              |
|      |             |                  |         |           |              |
|      |             |                  |         |           |              |
|      |             |                  |         |           |              |
|      |             |                  |         |           |              |
|      |             |                  |         |           |              |
|      |             |                  |         |           |              |
|      |             |                  |         |           |              |
|      |             |                  |         |           |              |
|      |             |                  |         |           |              |

# EVENING REFLECTION

*Sometimes the weight we need to lose isn't in our bodies, but in our thoughts.*

| HOW I FELT | 1 (DISSATISFIED) | 2 | 3 (SO-SO) | 4 | 5 (ON FIRE!) |
|---|---|---|---|---|---|
| MOOD | | | | | |
| ENERGY | | | | | |
| BLOOD SUGAR | | | | | |
| NUTRITION | | | | | |
| MINDSET | | | | | |

## TODAY I...

- ☐ EXERCISED
- ☐ MEDITATED
- ☐ EXPRESSED GRATITUDE
- ☐ SET GOALS FOR TODAY

- ☐ CHECKED MY SUGAR EVERY 2 HOURS
- ☐ WAS MINDFUL WHEN EATING
- ☐ MEAL PREPPED
- ☐ CARB COUNTED FOOD

- ☐ VISUALIZED DAY OF GOOD BLOOD SUGARS
- ☐ TOOK 10 DEEP BREATHS
- ☐ PRE-BOLUSED MEALS
- ☐ SPENT TIME WITH LOVED ONES

- ☐ TOOK A WALK OUTSIDE
- ☐ _____
- ☐ _____
- ☐ _____

EXERCISE: _____

WATER: ☐ ☐ ☐ ☐ ☐ ☐ ☐ ☐ ☐ ☐     TOTAL DAILY INSULIN: _____ UNITS

## THE NIGHT CAP

A PATTERN I RECOGNIZED WAS...

_____

_____

TOMORROW I WANT TO FOCUS MORE ON...

_____

_____

TODAY I CELEBRATE MYSELF BECAUSE...

_____

_____

# MORNING WORK IN | DATE: _____ S / M / T / W / T / F / S

## MINDSET PREP

I AM... _____

ONE THING I'M GRATEFUL FOR IS...

_____

ONE THING I DIDN'T DO YESTERDAY, BUT I WILL DO TODAY...

_____

## DAILY LOG

| TIME | BLOOD SUGAR | OUT OF RANGE (x) | INSULIN | C / F / P | NOTES / FOOD |
|------|-------------|------------------|---------|-----------|--------------|
|      |             |                  |         |           |              |
|      |             |                  |         |           |              |
|      |             |                  |         |           |              |
|      |             |                  |         |           |              |
|      |             |                  |         |           |              |
|      |             |                  |         |           |              |
|      |             |                  |         |           |              |
|      |             |                  |         |           |              |
|      |             |                  |         |           |              |
|      |             |                  |         |           |              |

# EVENING REFLECTION | "I am more than my scars." – Andrew Davidson

| HOW I FELT | 1 (DISSATISFIED) | 2 | 3 (SO-SO) | 4 | 5 (ON FIRE!) |
|---|---|---|---|---|---|
| MOOD | | | | | |
| ENERGY | | | | | |
| BLOOD SUGAR | | | | | |
| NUTRITION | | | | | |
| MINDSET | | | | | |

## TODAY I...

- ☐ EXERCISED
- ☐ CHECKED MY SUGAR EVERY 2 HOURS
- ☐ VISUALIZED DAY OF GOOD BLOOD SUGARS
- ☐ TOOK A WALK OUTSIDE

- ☐ MEDITATED
- ☐ WAS MINDFUL WHEN EATING
- ☐ TOOK 10 DEEP BREATHS
- ☐ _____

- ☐ EXPRESSED GRATITUDE
- ☐ MEAL PREPPED
- ☐ PRE-BOLUSED MEALS
- ☐ _____

- ☐ SET GOALS FOR TODAY
- ☐ CARB COUNTED FOOD
- ☐ SPENT TIME WITH LOVED ONES
- ☐ _____

EXERCISE: _____

WATER: ☐ ☐ ☐ ☐ ☐ ☐ ☐ ☐ ☐ ☐     TOTAL DAILY INSULIN: _____ UNITS

## THE NIGHT CAP

A PATTERN I RECOGNIZED WAS...

_____

_____

TOMORROW I WANT TO FOCUS MORE ON...

_____

_____

TODAY I CELEBRATE MYSELF BECAUSE...

_____

_____

# MORNING WORK IN
DATE: _____ S / M / T / W / T / F / S

## MINDSET PREP
I AM... _____

ONE THING I'M GRATEFUL FOR IS...

_____

ONE THING I DIDN'T DO YESTERDAY, BUT I WILL DO TODAY...

_____

## DAILY LOG

| TIME | BLOOD SUGAR | OUT OF RANGE (x) | INSULIN | C / F / P | NOTES / FOOD |
|------|-------------|------------------|---------|-----------|--------------|
|      |             |                  |         |           |              |
|      |             |                  |         |           |              |
|      |             |                  |         |           |              |
|      |             |                  |         |           |              |
|      |             |                  |         |           |              |
|      |             |                  |         |           |              |
|      |             |                  |         |           |              |
|      |             |                  |         |           |              |
|      |             |                  |         |           |              |
|      |             |                  |         |           |              |

# EVENING REFLECTION

**JOURNAL PROMPT:**
In what moments do you feel most alive?

| HOW I FELT | 1<br>(DISSATISFIED) | 2 | 3<br>(SO-SO) | 4 | 5<br>(ON FIRE!) |
|---|---|---|---|---|---|
| MOOD | | | | | |
| ENERGY | | | | | |
| BLOOD SUGAR | | | | | |
| NUTRITION | | | | | |
| MINDSET | | | | | |

## TODAY I...

- [ ] EXERCISED
- [ ] MEDITATED
- [ ] EXPRESSED GRATITUDE
- [ ] SET GOALS FOR TODAY

- [ ] CHECKED MY SUGAR EVERY 2 HOURS
- [ ] WAS MINDFUL WHEN EATING
- [ ] MEAL PREPPED
- [ ] CARB COUNTED FOOD

- [ ] VISUALIZED DAY OF GOOD BLOOD SUGARS
- [ ] TOOK 10 DEEP BREATHS
- [ ] PRE-BOLUSED MEALS
- [ ] SPENT TIME WITH LOVED ONES

- [ ] TOOK A WALK OUTSIDE
- [ ] _____
- [ ] _____
- [ ] _____

EXERCISE: _____

WATER: ⬜ ⬜ ⬜ ⬜ ⬜ ⬜ ⬜ ⬜ ⬜ ⬜      TOTAL DAILY INSULIN: _____ UNITS

## THE NIGHT CAP

A PATTERN I RECOGNIZED WAS...

_____

_____

TOMORROW I WANT TO FOCUS MORE ON...

_____

_____

TODAY I CELEBRATE MYSELF BECAUSE...

_____

_____

# MORNING WORK IN | DATE: _____ S / M / T / W / T / F / S

## MINDSET PREP

I AM... _____

ONE THING I'M GRATEFUL FOR IS...

_____

ONE THING I DIDN'T DO YESTERDAY, BUT I WILL DO TODAY...

_____

## DAILY LOG

| TIME | BLOOD SUGAR | OUT OF RANGE (x) | INSULIN | C / F / P | NOTES / FOOD |
|------|-------------|------------------|---------|-----------|--------------|
|      |             |                  |         |           |              |
|      |             |                  |         |           |              |
|      |             |                  |         |           |              |
|      |             |                  |         |           |              |
|      |             |                  |         |           |              |
|      |             |                  |         |           |              |
|      |             |                  |         |           |              |
|      |             |                  |         |           |              |
|      |             |                  |         |           |              |
|      |             |                  |         |           |              |

# EVENING REFLECTION | "To be good, and to do good, is all we have to do." – John Adams

| HOW I FELT | 1 (DISSATISFIED) | 2 | 3 (SO-SO) | 4 | 5 (ON FIRE!) |
|---|---|---|---|---|---|
| MOOD | | | | | |
| ENERGY | | | | | |
| BLOOD SUGAR | | | | | |
| NUTRITION | | | | | |
| MINDSET | | | | | |

## TODAY I...

- [ ] EXERCISED
- [ ] MEDITATED
- [ ] EXPRESSED GRATITUDE
- [ ] SET GOALS FOR TODAY

- [ ] CHECKED MY SUGAR EVERY 2 HOURS
- [ ] WAS MINDFUL WHEN EATING
- [ ] MEAL PREPPED
- [ ] CARB COUNTED FOOD

- [ ] VISUALIZED DAY OF GOOD BLOOD SUGARS
- [ ] TOOK 10 DEEP BREATHS
- [ ] PRE-BOLUSED MEALS
- [ ] SPENT TIME WITH LOVED ONES

- [ ] TOOK A WALK OUTSIDE
- [ ] _____
- [ ] _____
- [ ] _____

EXERCISE: _____

WATER: ▯ ▯ ▯ ▯ ▯ ▯ ▯ ▯ ▯ ▯     TOTAL DAILY INSULIN: _____ UNITS

## THE NIGHT CAP

A PATTERN I RECOGNIZED WAS...

_____

_____

TOMORROW I WANT TO FOCUS MORE ON...

_____

_____

TODAY I CELEBRATE MYSELF BECAUSE...

_____

_____

# MORNING WORK IN

DATE: _____ S / M / T / W / T / F / S

I AM... _____

ONE THING I'M GRATEFUL FOR IS...

_____

ONE THING I DIDN'T DO YESTERDAY, BUT I WILL DO TODAY...

_____

## DAILY LOG

| TIME | BLOOD SUGAR | OUT OF RANGE (x) | INSULIN | C / F / P | NOTES / FOOD |
|------|-------------|------------------|---------|-----------|--------------|
|      |             |                  |         |           |              |
|      |             |                  |         |           |              |
|      |             |                  |         |           |              |
|      |             |                  |         |           |              |
|      |             |                  |         |           |              |
|      |             |                  |         |           |              |
|      |             |                  |         |           |              |
|      |             |                  |         |           |              |
|      |             |                  |         |           |              |
|      |             |                  |         |           |              |

# EVENING REFLECTION | "Pain + Reflection equals Progress." – Ray Dalio

| HOW I FELT | 1 (DISSATISFIED) | 2 | 3 (SO-SO) | 4 | 5 (ON FIRE!) |
|---|---|---|---|---|---|
| MOOD | | | | | |
| ENERGY | | | | | |
| BLOOD SUGAR | | | | | |
| NUTRITION | | | | | |
| MINDSET | | | | | |

## TODAY I...

☐ EXERCISED  ☐ CHECKED MY SUGAR EVERY 2 HOURS  ☐ VISUALIZED DAY OF GOOD BLOOD SUGARS  ☐ TOOK A WALK OUTSIDE

☐ MEDITATED  ☐ WAS MINDFUL WHEN EATING  ☐ TOOK 10 DEEP BREATHS  ☐ _____

☐ EXPRESSED GRATITUDE  ☐ MEAL PREPPED  ☐ PRE-BOLUSED MEALS  ☐ _____

☐ SET GOALS FOR TODAY  ☐ CARB COUNTED FOOD  ☐ SPENT TIME WITH LOVED ONES  ☐ _____

EXERCISE: _____

WATER: ☐ ☐ ☐ ☐ ☐ ☐ ☐ ☐ ☐ ☐        TOTAL DAILY INSULIN: _____ UNITS

## THE NIGHT CAP

A PATTERN I RECOGNIZED WAS...

_____

_____

TOMORROW I WANT TO FOCUS MORE ON...

_____

_____

TODAY I CELEBRATE MYSELF BECAUSE...

_____

_____

# MORNING WORK IN | DATE: _____ S / M / T / W / T / F / S

## MINDSET PREP

I AM... _____

ONE THING I'M GRATEFUL FOR IS...

_____

ONE THING I DIDN'T DO YESTERDAY, BUT I WILL DO TODAY...

_____

## DAILY LOG

| TIME | BLOOD SUGAR | OUT OF RANGE (x) | INSULIN | C / F / P | NOTES / FOOD |
|------|-------------|------------------|---------|-----------|--------------|
|      |             |                  |         |           |              |
|      |             |                  |         |           |              |
|      |             |                  |         |           |              |
|      |             |                  |         |           |              |
|      |             |                  |         |           |              |
|      |             |                  |         |           |              |
|      |             |                  |         |           |              |
|      |             |                  |         |           |              |
|      |             |                  |         |           |              |
|      |             |                  |         |           |              |

# EVENING REFLECTION

"Nothing ever goes away until it has taught us what we need to know." – Pema Chödrön

| HOW I FELT | 1 (DISSATISFIED) | 2 | 3 (SO-SO) | 4 | 5 (ON FIRE!) |
|---|---|---|---|---|---|
| MOOD | | | | | |
| ENERGY | | | | | |
| BLOOD SUGAR | | | | | |
| NUTRITION | | | | | |
| MINDSET | | | | | |

## TODAY I...

- ☐ EXERCISED
- ☐ CHECKED MY SUGAR EVERY 2 HOURS
- ☐ VISUALIZED DAY OF GOOD BLOOD SUGARS
- ☐ TOOK A WALK OUTSIDE

- ☐ MEDITATED
- ☐ WAS MINDFUL WHEN EATING
- ☐ TOOK 10 DEEP BREATHS
- ☐ _____

- ☐ EXPRESSED GRATITUDE
- ☐ MEAL PREPPED
- ☐ PRE-BOLUSED MEALS
- ☐ _____

- ☐ SET GOALS FOR TODAY
- ☐ CARB COUNTED FOOD
- ☐ SPENT TIME WITH LOVED ONES
- ☐ _____

EXERCISE: _____

WATER: ☐ ☐ ☐ ☐ ☐ ☐ ☐ ☐ ☐ ☐     TOTAL DAILY INSULIN: _____ UNITS

## THE NIGHT CAP

A PATTERN I RECOGNIZED WAS...

_____

_____

TOMORROW I WANT TO FOCUS MORE ON...

_____

_____

TODAY I CELEBRATE MYSELF BECAUSE...

_____

_____

# MORNING WORK IN | DATE: _____ S / M / T / W / T / F / S

## MINDSET PREP

I AM... _____

ONE THING I'M GRATEFUL FOR IS...

_____

ONE THING I DIDN'T DO YESTERDAY, BUT I WILL DO TODAY...

_____

## DAILY LOG

| TIME | BLOOD SUGAR | OUT OF RANGE (x) | INSULIN | C / F / P | NOTES / FOOD |
|------|-------------|------------------|---------|-----------|--------------|
|      |             |                  |         |           |              |
|      |             |                  |         |           |              |
|      |             |                  |         |           |              |
|      |             |                  |         |           |              |
|      |             |                  |         |           |              |
|      |             |                  |         |           |              |
|      |             |                  |         |           |              |
|      |             |                  |         |           |              |
|      |             |                  |         |           |              |
|      |             |                  |         |           |              |

# EVENING REFLECTION

"Fearlessness is not avoiding the ups + downs of life:
It's sitting with them, listening, feeling, bowing to them,
and then moving forward." – Waylon Lewis

| HOW I FELT | 1 (DISSATISFIED) | 2 | 3 (SO-SO) | 4 | 5 (ON FIRE!) |
|---|---|---|---|---|---|
| MOOD | | | | | |
| ENERGY | | | | | |
| BLOOD SUGAR | | | | | |
| NUTRITION | | | | | |
| MINDSET | | | | | |

## TODAY I...

☐ EXERCISED

☐ MEDITATED

☐ EXPRESSED GRATITUDE

☐ SET GOALS FOR TODAY

☐ CHECKED MY SUGAR EVERY 2 HOURS

☐ WAS MINDFUL WHEN EATING

☐ MEAL PREPPED

☐ CARB COUNTED FOOD

☐ VISUALIZED DAY OF GOOD BLOOD SUGARS

☐ TOOK 10 DEEP BREATHS

☐ PRE-BOLUSED MEALS

☐ SPENT TIME WITH LOVED ONES

☐ TOOK A WALK OUTSIDE

☐ _____

☐ _____

☐ _____

EXERCISE: _____

WATER: ▽ ▽ ▽ ▽ ▽ ▽ ▽ ▽ ▽ ▽      TOTAL DAILY INSULIN: _____ UNITS

## THE NIGHT CAP

A PATTERN I RECOGNIZED WAS...

_____

_____

TOMORROW I WANT TO FOCUS MORE ON...

_____

_____

TODAY I CELEBRATE MYSELF BECAUSE...

_____

_____

# MONTH 03 REVIEW + REFLECT

## SELF ASSESSMENT

1. What is your new A1C? _____

2. What is your average fasting blood sugar (waking up)? _____

3. My current basal insulin:

| TIME OF DAY | MY BASAL |
|---|---|
| 12:00am | |
| | |
| | |
| | |
| | |
| | |
| | |

4. My current Insulin: Carb Ratio/s:

| TIME OF DAY | MY ICR |
|---|---|
| 12:00am | |
| | |
| | |
| | |
| | |
| | |
| | |

5. My current Insulin Sensitivity Factor/s:

| TIME OF DAY | MY ISF |
|---|---|
| 12:00am | |
| | |
| | |
| | |
| | |
| | |
| | |

6. On a scale from 0-10, rate your happiness in each of the following areas:

_____ a.) Diabetes Management

_____ b.) Exercise

_____ c.) Sleep

_____ d.) Energy

_____ e.) Peace of Mind/Stress and Anxiety Management

_____ f.) Nutrition/Relationship with Food

_____ g.) Relationships with Family, Friends, and Co-Workers

_____ h.) Self Love/Acceptance

7. My target Blood Glucose:

_____

# MIND / BODY / SOUL

1. Compare the results of your happiness exercise on the previous page to your results of the exercise before you started this journal. What has changed? Which improvements are you most proud of?

_____

_____

_____

_____

2. What actions over the last three months have best served your blood sugar management?

_____

_____

_____

_____

3. What actions do you want to continue to maintain progress moving forward?

_____

_____

_____

_____

## DECIDE + CONQUER

Here's to you for working on yourself daily over the last three months! Regardless of what type of progress you've cultivated, know that you are strong, inspiring, resilient, and capable. Remember, T1D warriors never tap out. We never stop being challenged. We never stop growing. We see a problem, we find a solution. Decide and conquer. It's what you were born to do.

xo, Lauren

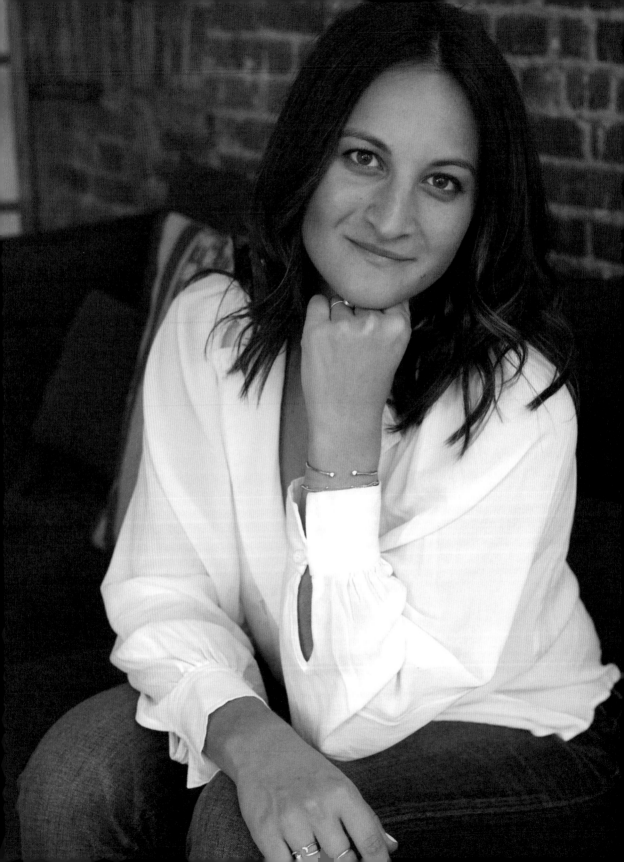

# ABOUT LAUREN

Lauren Bongiorno is a Diabetic Health Coach, Yoga instructor, author, wellness speaker, and former Division 1 Collegiate Athlete. At the age of 7, Lauren was diagnosed with Type 1 Diabetes, a condition that ultimately led her to finding her true passion and purpose in life. With the commitment to a holistic approach to health, Lauren educates, supports, and guides type 1 diabetics all around the globe in taking control of their diabetes by developing healthful habits and mindsets for the mind, body, and soul. Over the past few years, Lauren has become a voice in the online diabetic community through her Instagram page, @lauren_bongiorno. To connect with or learn more about Lauren, visit www.laurenbongiorno.com.

CONNECT WITH LAUREN
INSTAGRAM • @lauren_bongiorno
WEBSITE • www.laurenbongiorno.com

CONNECT WITH #myDHJ TRIBE

INSTAGRAM • @diabetichealthjournal
DECIDE & CONQUER FACEBOOK GROUP • https://www.facebook.com/groups/decideandconquerdiabetes/
WEBSITE • www.diabetichealthjournal.com